Pursuing Perfection

In *Pursuing Perfection*, authors Margo Maine and Joe Kelly explore the emotional, social and cultural factors behind the ongoing epidemic of disordered eating and body image despair in adult women at midlife and beyond. Written from a biopsychosocial and feminist perspective, *Pursuing Perfection* describes the many issues women encounter as they navigate a rapidly changing culture that promotes unhealthy standards for beauty and appearance. This updated and expanded edition (originally published as *The Body Myth: Adult Women and the Pressure to Be Perfect*) is a unique guide for anyone seeking practical tools and strategies for adult women looking to establish health and body acceptance.

Margo Maine, PhD, FAED, CEDS, has spent over 35 years treating a broad range of eating disorders and body image issues. In her West Hartford, Connecticut practice, she treats women of all ages, shapes, sizes, cultures, races and ethnicities. A lecturer, consultant and researcher, Dr. Maine is a senior editor of *Eating Disorders: The Journal of Treatment and Prevention*. Additionally, she is a founding member and Fellow of the Academy for Eating Disorders; former vice-president of the Eating Disorders Coalition for Research, Policy, and Action; a founder and senior advisor to the National Eating Disorders Association and the 2015 recipient of its Lifetime Achievement Award.

Joe Kelly is a best-selling author, editor, educator, father and grandfather in Emeryville, California. Formerly a Minnesota Public Radio regional News Director, he co-founded the international, award-winning, girl-edited magazine *New Moon Girls* and the national advocacy nonprofit Dads and Daughters®. Kelly helps health and education professionals to mobilize and utilize their clients' and students' male loved ones as resources and also coaches men and women with family members suffering from eating disorders and/or addiction.

Pursuing Perfection

Eating Disorders, Body Myths and
Women at Midlife and Beyond

**Margo Maine, PhD, FAED, CEDS
and Joe Kelly**

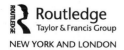

Routledge
Taylor & Francis Group

NEW YORK AND LONDON

First published 2016
by Routledge
711 Third Avenue, New York, NY 10017

and by Routledge
2 Park Square, Milton Park, Abingdon, Oxon, OX14 4RN

Routledge is an imprint of the Taylor & Francis Group, an informa business

Library of Congress Cataloging in Publication Data
Names: Maine, Margo, author. | Kelly, Joe, 1954- author.
Title: Pursuing perfection : eating disorders, body myths, and women at midlife and beyond / Margo Maine, Ph.D. and Joe Kelly.
Other titles: Body myth
Description: New York, NY : Routledge, 2016. | Revision of: Body myth / Margo Maine and Joe Kelly. 2005. | Includes bibliographical references and index.
Identifiers: LCCN 2015048763 (print) | LCCN 2016006509 (ebook) | ISBN 9781138890718 (hbk : alk. paper) | ISBN 9781138890725 (pbk : alk. paper) | ISBN 9781315710099 (ebk)
Subjects: LCSH: Eating disorders in women.
Classification: LCC RC552.E18 M32 2016 (print) | LCC RC552.E18 (ebook) | DDC 616.85/260082--dc23
LC record available at http://lccn.loc.gov/2015048763

ISBN: 978-1-138-89071-8 (hbk)
ISBN: 978-1-138-89072-5 (pbk)
ISBN: 978-1-315-71009-9 (ebk)

Typeset in Sabon
by HWA Text and Data Management, London

Acknowledgments

Many people helped us to discuss this book, explore its imperfections, and refine its ideas. We particularly thank Carol Dohanyos, Lin Druschel, Beth McGilley, Adrienne Ressler, Gail R. Schoenbach, Kitty Westin and other friends who prefer to remain unnamed for deepening our understanding of how women experience their bodies in our culture, even when they do not have eating or body image disorders.

Our colleagues Michael Levine, PhD, Rosalie Maggio and Diane Mickley, MD, were a tremendous help in tracking down and clarifying important data in the book.

We are grateful to Robin Dellabough for helping to launch this book and especially blessed to have Christopher Teja as our editor for this project. We encountered surprising resistance to this book in some publishing circles, where people seemed somehow threatened by its simple message. However, Robin understood the importance of what we wrote, as did Chris and his associates at Routledge. We deeply appreciate their collaboration, support and commitment to educating the world about the tenacity of eating disorders in adult women's lives today.

Many other colleagues listened, taught and encouraged us through this and previous projects, including Hollie Ainbinder, Michael Berrett, Francie Berg, Bruce Brody, Joan Jacobs Brumberg, Doug Bunnell, Pamela Carlton, Jeanine Cogan, Leigh Cohn, Carolyn Costin, Bill Davis, Steve Emmett, Sandra Friedman, Kari Fox, Mary Gee, Judi Goldstein, the late Lynn Grefe, Lindsey Hall, David Herzog, Craig Johnson, Matt Kaler, Marilyn Karr, Kathy Kater, Ann Kearney-Cooke, Michael Kieschnick, Jean Kilbourne, Sondra Kronberg, Susan Linn, Lise Lunge-Larsen, Paula Levine, Sam Menaged, Lyn Mikel Brown, Mary Pabst, Judith Ruskay Rabinor, Stacy Saindon, Karen Samuels, Meri Shadley, Jane Shure, Brenda Alpert Sigall, Anita Sinicrope Maier, Mary Tantillo, Sean Taylor, Rob Weinstein and Dina Zeckhausen.

Our spouses George and Nancy continue to encourage our passion for writing, even though it often takes us away from them (or maybe because it gives them a break from us!). Either way, we are deeply grateful to them for their support—and for so much more.

Contents

To my brave patients who decide it's never too late to break out of the prison of perfectionism and make peace with their bodies. Bravo! You are amazing and inspiring. Thank you for trusting me to help you on your journey.

MM

To Heather Henderson and the countless people she helped in her too-short life.

JK

Finally we thank Margo's adult patients, who have been brave enough to ask for help and gutsy enough to change their relationships with their bodies and their worlds. You are an inspiration to us and, through your contribution to *Pursuing Perfection*, an inspiration to women and men you will never know. Thank you.

West Hartford, Connecticut and Emeryville, California
April, 2016

Introduction

A dedication to perfection means that we are doomed always to be just a heartbeat away—from exposure. Perfection is unchanging; lives are ongoing.[1]

Joy Browne

In the relatively short history of eating disorders treatment, the overwhelming majority of patients and clients have been young women between their teens and 20s. In most cases, a young woman's mother makes the first calls for help, arranging therapy, medical attention and other treatment for her daughter.

Adult women still make those initial calls to an eating disorder or body image professional. But, far more frequently, these women call to get help not for their daughters, but for *themselves*.

In recent years, media outlets have regularly asked me to discuss the growing number of women over 30 seeking treatment for eating disorders.[2] I explain that women of all ages do indeed struggle with eating disorders and body image issues; it's not as if adult women are immunized from these problems or magically outgrow them. Each time a news story appears, I receive dozens of calls from additional reports and producers. I also hear from many ordinary women saying, "This is every woman's secret. It's about time we started talking about it."

This buzz of media interest reflects the mounting number of women in their 30s, 40s, 50s, 60s and even older who suffer with seriously disordered eating or body image problems. A major US treatment program, the Renfrew Center, reports a truly massive shift: one-third of its residential patients are now over 30. Between 2001 and 2011, Renfrew logged a 42 percent increase in women over 35 seeking their services.[3]

This phenomenon isn't isolated to one treatment agency. Statistics on admissions for inpatient eating disorders treatment between 1999 and 2009 showed the greatest increase among older patients, with women over age 45 accounting for a full 25 percent of those admissions.[4] In today's United States of America, the prevalence of disordered eating behaviors and serious weight and shape concerns among women over 50 is now slightly higher than the prevalence of breast cancer (13 percent[5] vs. 12 percent[6]).

In other words, we have both clinical research and population-based surveys documenting a major public health issue: the epidemic of body image and eating issues that plague women (and men) of all ages.

Whenever I speak about these issues, I remind my listeners that "statistics are people with the tears wiped away."[7] On the outside, most adult women I treat seem successful in their careers, and appear to have their lives under control. They are wonderful, resourceful women with tremendous strengths.

Inside, however, they spiral through frightening and dreary stages of severe dieting, bingeing, purging and weight obsession, as they try to be perfect and meet our culture's appearance expectations. The pressure to be perfect leads them to a perfect problem: the deeply embedded (but mistaken) belief that our meaning, self-worth and value to others are (and ought to be) based on how our bodies appear, what we weigh, and what we eat.

> In order to go on living one must try to escape the death involved in perfection.[8]
>
> Hannah Arendt

Perfectionism comes with a hefty price tag, eating away at our emotional and physical well-being. Perfectionism makes it easy to succumb to the myths claiming that weight loss or a sculpted and "perfected" body will bring meaning and value to us. Cindy Ratzlaff and Kathy Kinney, authors of *Queen of Your Own Life: The Grown-up Woman's Guide to Claiming Happiness and Getting the Life You Deserve*, call perfectionism "the leading fatal disease among women 18 to 100."[9]

Ironically, the pressure to be perfect also undermines many gains made by women over the last century. According to Barnard College president Debora Spar, PhD, modern women have morphed feminism into perfectionism:

> I'm not entirely sure why, but I think one of the things that happened without anyone meaning for it to happen is that as we generationally all got excited with these tremendous opportunities that were being created for women, we kind of built a myth and an illusion around it. We not only thought that we would have all of these things at once, but that somehow we would glide into this life without really having to work very hard; without struggling, without failing, without getting depressed. And the result of that, sadly, is that when our lives (of course) become harder and become messier, we somehow feel like we failed.[10]

A 2011 Gallup-Healthways Well-Being Index shows that women aged 45 to 64 have the lowest well-being and highest stress of any age group or gender. In addition, as social worker Michelle Martin, PhD, writes:

> The study highlighted the fact that among a range of emotions experienced by these over-worked and under-appreciated women, the most pronounced was guilt. No matter how much they worked, no matter how thinly they were spread, no matter how caring, giving, and sacrificing (and no matter how damned good they looked while engaging in all of their service-related activities) it never felt like they were doing enough—there was always more they believed they could/should/needed to do.[11]

The pressure on women to pursue perfection does not discriminate by race, ethnicity, or age. Neither do eating disorders. Despite the common perception that minority women are unlikely to suffer from them, the multi-ethnic Study of Women's Health Across the Nation (SWAN) found that disordered eating was common in women aged 42 to 55—and evenly distributed across African-American, Hispanic and Caucasian populations.[12] Groundbreaking books like Becky Thompson's *A Hunger So Wide and So Deep*[13] and Stephanie Covington Armstrong's *Not All Black Girls Know How to Eat*[14] eloquently explain African-American women's struggle with abnormal eating attitudes and behaviors.

What's happening here? Eating disorders and body image despair aren't contagious or a matter of inverted heredity, spreading from young women to their mothers. Who are these adult women and why do they need help?

They may be women struggling with body image loathing that arose during their youth and never fully abated.

They may have suffered from an eating disorder in their teens or 20s, and pulled out of the downward spiral for decades, only to relapse when they are older.

They may have been preoccupied with food and weight for years, but are now incapacitated in maturity.

They may be women who, faced with the challenges of adulthood and loss of status in a youth-oriented world, develop eating obsessions or a distorted body image for the first time in their lives.

As adult women, we have come to live under the terms of a widely accepted perfection myth: that the answer to our life's meaning and challenges lies in our body's appearance. This book reveals why and how body image, appetite and hunger have become so central to women's lives, exposing the deep pain and disruption they cause.

But I also make clear how adult women with eating disorders and other serious body image problems are truly *different* from their adolescent counterparts. The misperception that these problems are limited only to teenagers often causes adult women with body and food issues to feel even more abnormal and alone than they would otherwise. Many see no place to turn, and no sign that their peers share what seems like a "girl's" problem. Shame that she hasn't gotten beyond such problems isolates a woman, which in turn makes it more difficult to seek and accept help.

I wrote *Pursuing Perfection* as a practical, jargon-free guide to recognizing the signs of eating disorders and self-loathing—and understanding how to get help. The book has concrete strategies to address other related problems (like yo-yo dieting, problem eating and body image distress) that also sap sustenance from adult women and distort their lives.

For too long, body image despair, and the perfectionistic myths that feed it, have remained a miserable secret and source of shame that adult women are afraid to reveal to each other, or even to themselves.

Admitting that perfectionism has become a destructive force in our lives would mean admitting our imperfections: a fundamental Catch 22. Paradoxically, once women break that silence, we can see how perfectionism and body hatred actually keep us from confronting the true challenges of our adult life like loss, guilt, regret, aging and mortality. Elizabeth Gilbert, an astute observer of women's lives today, describes perfectionism as "the haute couture, high-end version of fear ... It's just fear in really good shoes ... But it's still fear."15

So as you read this book, take time to ponder what fears underlie, and are camouflaged by, your perfectionism.

Pursuing Perfection helps women to rethink how we look at our own bodies, reshape how other people think about adult women, and discover positive alternatives for measuring women's self-worth. It taps great hope and inspiration in the voices of adult women who are overcoming body image despair and eating disorders every day.

Pursuing Perfection is also a "biblio-therapy" resource we can share and discuss with other people, or use as a support in the privacy of our homes. Together, its stories can help women, men and our world discard body myths, get off the body image merry-go-round and to take the first steps toward recovering the rich and imperfect lives each of us is meant to live.

Instead of women venturing to "perfect" our bodies' appearance, I want us to embrace the adventure of this flawed, mysterious and beautiful world. May this book be your first step on that adventure.

Notes

1 *The Nine Fantasies That Will Ruin Your Life and the Eight Realities That Will Save You* (New York: Harmony Books, 2010) p. 22.
2 E.g., *Katie Couric Show*, aired May 14, 2013; "Eating disorders: Not just for the young," CNN, posted June 27, 2012. See www.cnn.com/2012/06/26/health/mental-health/eating-disorders-not-just-for-young/ (retrieved September 13, 2015); "Eating disorders affect adults, too," San Antonio Express-News. See www.expressnews.com/lifestyle/health-family/article/Eating-disorders-affect-

adults-too-6298718.php (retrieved September 13, 2015); and "An excerpt from Mika Brzezinski's *Obsessed*," MSNBC. See www.msnbc.com/morning-joe/excerpt-mika-brzezinskis-obsessed (retrieved September 13, 2015).

3 Personal correspondence with Margo Maine.

4 Yafu Zhao and William Encinosa (2011), "An update on hospitalizations for eating disorders, 1999 to 2009." *Healthcare Cost and Utilization Project (HCUP) Statistical Brief #120* (Rockville, MD: US Agency for Health Care Policy and Research).

5 Danielle A. Gagne, Ann Von Holle, Kimberly A. Brownley, Cristin D. Runfola, Sara Hofmeier, Kateland E. Branch and Cynthia M. Bulik (2012) "Eating disorder symptoms and weight and shape concerns in a large web-based convenience sample of women ages 50 and above: Results of the gender and body image (GABI) study." *International Journal of Eating Disorders*, 45 (7), 832–844.

6 National Cancer Institute, "Breast cancer risk in American women." See www.cancer.gov/cancertopics/types/breast/risk-fact-sheet (retrieved September 13, 2015).

7 Paul Brodeur, *Outrageous Misconduct: The Asbestos Industry on Trial* (New York: Pantheon, 1985).

8 *Rahel Varnhagen: The Life of a Jewess* translated from the German by Richard and Clara Winston, Publications of the Leo Baeck Institute of Jews from Germany (London: East and West Library, 1958) p. 129.

9 The Massachusetts Conference for Women, "Perfectionism: The leading fatal disease among women 18 to 100." See www.maconferenceforwomen.org/perfectionism-leading-fatal-disease-among-women-18-100/ (retrieved September 13, 2015).

10 Kelly Wallace, "Ladies, stop trying to be perfect!" Cable News Network (CNN). Posted October 2, 2013, www.cnn.com/2013/10/02/living/parents-perfectionism-tips-debora-spar/ (retrieved September 13, 2015).

11 "5 things women with perfectionistic guilt need to hear." Posted March 19, 2015, www.huffingtonpost.com/michelle-martin/things-women-with-perfectionistic-guilt-need-to-hear_b_6828820.html (retrieved September 13, 2015).

12 Marsha D. Marcus, Joyce T. Bromberger, Hsiao-Lan Wei, Charlotte Brown and Howard M. Kravitz (2007) "Prevalence and selected correlates of eating disorder symptoms among a multiethnic community sample of midlife women." *Annals of Behavioral Medicine*, 33, 269–277.

13 Minneapolis, MN: University of Minnesota Press, 1996.

14 Chicago, IL: Chicago Review Press, 2009.

15 "Perfectionism is 'just fear in really good shoes'." *Huffington Post Own Videos*, posted October 2, 2014, www.huffingtonpost.com/2014/10/02/elizabeth-gilbert-oprah-root-of-every-problem_n_5914412.html (retrieved September 18, 2015).

Glossary

A Word about Words

When discussing this book's complex and emotionally charged issues, we face the problem of what terms to use. For example, the word "diet" can have different, almost opposite, meanings. Most of us think of diet as "a plan for restricting the amount of food someone eats." But diet can also describe the simple act of eating itself, or the common food and drink for a person or culture—for example, "Milk is a staple of the American diet."

So, to cut down on the confusion, I've come up with simple descriptions below of what *I* mean when I use essential terms in *this* book.

Adult: a person who has reached physical growth, development and maturity. In this book, "adult" means people over 30, "young adult" means people 20–29 years old, "teen" covers ages 13 to 19, and "child" is anyone younger than 13.

Aging: the normal process that every person (including infants) undergoes daily. In this book, aging is not a disparaging or negative concept—it is a fact.

Appetite: the psychologically triggered craving for food (as opposed to the physiological trigger of hunger, see below); a healthy desire to eat food and drink liquids. Appetite comes from the Latin word *appetere*, meaning "to long for" or "to strive after."

Appetites: the psychological desire to feel, experience, take in, accept, deserve, connect, risk, comfort, be comforted and be free. Becoming fully adult means addressing these "metaphorical" hungers. As Caroline Knapp writes in her book *Appetites*: "[A] woman's individual preoccupation with weight often serves as a mask for other, more intricate sources of discomfort, the state of one's waistline being easier to contemplate than the state of one's soul."[1]

Bingeing and purging: a dangerous practice of eating beyond the point of being or feeling full (bingeing) and then forcing the food out of our body (purging) with vomiting, laxatives, diuretics, etc. People binge and purge in an attempt to relieve emotional stress and/or pain.

Body: the physical home of the heart, mind, movement, passion, searching, satiation.

Body image: one's personal perception and judgment of the size, shape, weight and any other aspect of her body that relates to body appearance—from hair style and make-up to skin tone and clothing. Body image is different from what the body itself actually looks like to an outside observer. Notice how there is no innate negative connotation in this definition.

Body myths: commonly held misconceptions about appearance, weight, food and how the body works. For example, the myth that dieting is a successful strategy for losing weight.

Culture: our collective way of life: all the ideas, objects and ways of doing things created by the group. It includes arts, beliefs, customs, institutions, inventions, language, media, technology and traditions. We shape the culture through the attitudes and behaviors we encourage—and those we allow to pass unchallenged. Culture also shapes us from childhood through old age.

Diet: most people use "diet" to mean a method of restricting food intake in an attempt to lose weight. That meaning has subsumed the dictionary definition of the word: the food and drink that an individual or group usually eats. In this book, I will use "diet" to mean "dieting to lose weight" or restricted intake of food. Dieting to lose weight can easily disrupt the hunger-cue system (see "hunger" later) and lead to other serious problems.

Disordered eating/problem eating: aberrant behaviors (like cyclical dieting) that tend to break the natural connection between eating and nutrition. While disordered eating may not rise to the diagnosis of a full-blown eating disorder, it does cause both psychological and physical harm. It can also lead to eating disorders. Even short periods of disordered eating can send a woman into emotional tailspins as she wastes precious time and energy obsessing about food and weight. Disordered eating puts metabolism and brain chemistry out of balance, causing depression, anxiety and irritability.

Eating disorders: complex, diagnosable and *real* illnesses triggered by behavioral, emotional, physical, psychological, spiritual, interpersonal and cultural factors. People with eating disorders often use food and the control of food in an attempt to compensate for feelings and emotions that seem painful and overwhelming. Eating disorders ultimately damage a person's physical and emotional health, and can lead to premature death. They include anorexia nervosa (which has the highest mortality rate of any mental illness), bulimia nervosa, binge eating disorder (BED) and variations of these, called Other Specified Feeding or Eating Disorder (OSFED).

Exercise abuse: exercise is abusive when a person: cancels or avoids other activities and obligations in order to exercise; exercises incessantly, whether ill, injured, or exhausted; or bases her self-worth on how much she exercises. Exercise is abusive when one always pushes herself to do more; becomes angry, anxious, or agitated when she cannot exercise; or when she uses it to compensate for calories eaten rather than for health and enjoyment.

Fat (substance): a noun that describes cells in the human body (as well as in other animals and some plants) made primarily of carbon, hydrogen and oxygen. Fats are essential for human survival, especially a female's ability to give birth, lactate and pass through menopause. Fat cells are compounds of several acids, and do not dissolve in water.

Fat (shape): an adjective (like short, tall, red-headed) that describes someone's body. A fat body is larger and fleshier than a thin body. Our current culture uses the word "fat" to insult or belittle, but during history (and in other cultures), the fat figure has deeply attractive and sensual connotations (see the paintings of Renoir). This book uses "fat" (rather than "overweight") as a purely descriptive, nonjudgmental adjective. "Overweight" is an inexact term that reinforces harmful body myths about weight and diet.

Health: the state of one's body and mind. Weight and body shape *may* be signs of good or poor health, but our culture's body myths tends to make them the primary or *only* signs of health. Contrary to popular belief, one can be thin and not healthy, or one can be fit, fat and in excellent health. Genetics, lifestyle, activity level and nutritional intake predict health much more accurately than weight does.

Hunger: the physiologically triggered craving for food; pain or discomfort in the stomach which is a cue for a person to eat (as opposed to the psychological trigger of appetite; see above). Hunger is the body's response to its need for nutrition and fuel.

Midlife: the time of life when a person becomes more conscious of her mortality, and experiences major life changes like children moving away from home or a parent dying. Midlife usually refers to our 40s and 50s. The average woman in the US lives 81.2 years, so her actual "midlife point" is 40.6 years.[2]

Normal eating: flexible and natural eating. It is a *range* of different behaviors at different times and in different circumstances. Normal eating responds to internal cues regarding hunger or emotional needs (wanting a comfort food or celebrating an event with a favorite food). Normal eating also responds to external cues such as a food's availability, aroma, appearance, or religious and family rituals (like weddings and funerals). Normal eating includes sometimes eating too much just because we feel like it! When eating normally, a person is not afraid of food.

Normal weight: a weight *range* resulting from a combination of nature and nurture. Weight is one measure of our body's relationship to gravity. Our weight is affected by a wide range of factors, including genetics, early experiences with food (are we fed too much? Too little? Are we taught to listen to our hunger, or expected to eat to satisfy our caregivers?), later experiences (especially illnesses or certain medications) and lifestyle. As with so many things, when it comes to weight, the whole is greater than the sum of its parts. If we eat well, are physically active, and don't have a chronic illness, then we will settle into a weight *range* that shifts over the course of life and continually reflects our genetic heritage.

Nutrition: how a person eats and how her body uses food once it is ingested. Nutrition also means supplying or receiving food for nourishment. Both nutrition and nourishment come from the Latin word for "to feed" and refer to making something grow or keeping it alive and well with food.

Thin: an adjective (like short, tall, red-headed) that describes a body that is less wide and fleshy than a fat body. As with "fat," this book uses "thin" as a purely descriptive, nonjudgmental adjective.

A Note about Names

Throughout this book, you'll read stories of adult women struggling with eating disorders, body image and other issues. All of these women are real, but their names and some of their identifying characteristics have been changed to protect their privacy.

Notes

1 *Appetites: Why Women Want* (Berkeley, CA: Counterpoint, 2004) p. 17.
2 Centers for Disease Control (2014) "Health, United States, 2014" (Washington, DC: U.S. Government Printing Office) p. 83. See www.cdc. gov/nchs/data/hus/hus14.pdf#015 (retrieved September 13, 2015).

1　The Changing Shape of Womanhood

The thing that is really hard, and really amazing, is giving up on being perfect and beginning the work of becoming yourself.[1]

Anna Quindlen

Adult women today suffer from endless pressures to do and be everything … perfectly. This Pursuit of Perfection is a fast track to:

- anxiety
- depression
- substance abuse
- compulsive behaviors
- a deep sense of shame
- a deep sense of inadequacy.

The pursuit of perfection also paves a path to eating disorders for women in their 30s, 40s, 50s and beyond—despite the widespread misconception that these deadly illnesses are merely an adolescent "phase."

Even after reaching "middle age," many women continue their pursuit of a perfect body—relentlessly scrutinizing every ounce of fat, every morsel consumed, every imaginable and imagined flaw. Eating disorders are an unsurprising result of this scrutiny. They reinforce the prison of perfectionism, hide the keys, and proceed to destroy lives.

Jennifer's Story

Consider my client Jennifer, an attractive, successful and well-liked woman in her 40s. She is a Super Mom, Super Employee, Super Wife, Super Daughter, Super Sister, Super Aunt, Super Niece, Super Cousin, Super Volunteer, Super Neighbor and Super Friend. People are awed by her; she always looks "perfect," pretty, stylish and thin—like she has it all. But inside, this Superwoman is exhausted, depressed, and running on empty.

Jennifer and her husband Bill have a preteen daughter and teen son. Bill is deeply involved in his work and is a high profile volunteer in their community. He isn't very available with his time or emotions, so Jennifer manages most details of family life, including schedules for Bill, their marriage, their kids, her parents and Bill's parents.

Her parents and in-laws are getting older, and starting to have health problems. They all rely on Jennifer's aid. She wants to help them more, and feels guilty if she can't be there for them. In fact, Jennifer feels besieged while trying to hold the home front together in the complex, accelerating rush of 21st century family life, while also being expected to work outside the home. Despite the burdens, Jennifer projects a cheerful attitude, seeming to easily juggle her whole family's needs and to manage her career.

Jennifer doesn't know how to stop "doing everything" for fear that her world will fly apart and she'll let down the people she loves. While she knows it's impossible, Jennifer keeps trying to be perfect and rarely asks for help. She tends to be a "control junkie," attempting to micromanage the minutia of her life and her family's life because she feels so little command over the larger forces affecting her world and her family.

Jennifer's body is also complex, changing its rhythms and shape as she moves through midlife. Despite this, she has been led to believe (by her upbringing, the culture and the media) that she can—and should—control her body's shape, weight, appearance and aging.

So when she feels overrun by life's requirements and uncertainties, Jennifer fights determinedly to make her body obey her commands. This helps her feel more in control than when she faces the overwhelming demands of her overall situation, the ambiguity she feels about her life and the daily comments she gets from other people about her body.

Years ago Jennifer learned to assess her self-worth on the bathroom scale, and to translate her negative emotions into what body image educator Sandra S. Friedman calls "the language of fat."[2] That's why Jennifer has been dieting and struggling with body image issues since she was a teenager. Adult stresses easily rekindle those struggles. Like most women with eating disorders, Jennifer kept her problem well hidden and no one seemed to notice.

Because she had difficulty getting pregnant, Jennifer had fertility treatment, which made her gain weight. Pregnancies brought even more weight concern and she dieted severely after each birth. Jennifer feels that postpartum crash diets were essential to keep Bill interested in her. Jennifer "changes" her body rather than explore the mistrust simmering just below the surface of her marriage. It is scary to ask why she fears that Bill would leave her if she wasn't physically "attractive" enough.

Her postpartum diet goal was returning to her original weight, but she overshot each target, becoming thinner after pregnancy than she was before it. She likes how people frequently compliment her appearance and emphatically praise her weight loss. But while her OB/GYN never addressed it, she still worries about how and why her periods became wildly irregular after her second postpartum diet. Now that she's entering menopause, Jennifer feels even less control of her body and everything else in her life. Afraid that she will gain weight during menopause, she restricts her food intake more strictly, and combines periodic vomiting with hours of intense daily exercise to fight the pounds.

Jennifer's façade is beginning to crack. The weight is coming off, but she isn't getting the same esteem fix that dieting used to deliver. Instead of feeling more satisfied, Jennifer feels more anxious. She's always been very close to her kids, but now feels left out of their adolescent lives. Her son Jerry is less communicative and she deeply misses their former closeness. Her daughter Mandy reminds Jennifer of herself at age 12: rigid, competitive and always pushing herself. The familiar way Mandy criticizes her body and obsesses about dieting frightens Jennifer. She is afraid Mandy will replicate Jennifer's own decades of body struggle.

Watching Mandy, Jennifer decides she can't leave this painful legacy to her daughter. Jennifer admits to herself that she has some kind of problem, but is ashamed that it has lingered so long into adulthood. Convinced that body image obsession is a teenager's problem, she thinks she should be over it. But finally, Jennifer gathers the courage to bring her concerns to her gynecologist at her next checkup.

Before she can even mention her concerns, however, the nurse enthusiastically compliments Jennifer on her appearance and asks how she was able to keep all that weight off and look so good. The doctor is just as flattering when he enters the exam room. Feeling misunderstood and confused, she never asks him for help or tells the truth about her fluctuating periods and the dangerous ways she manages her weight. Jennifer goes home frightened, ashamed, hopeless and uncertain what to do next. From what people tell her, she looks "better and better" on the outside, but she feels worse and worse inside her "perfect" little body.

The Shape of Womanhood

For Jennifer and many other women, the body becomes the answer to all angst, appearing to provide concrete answers to abstract questions such as "How am I faring as a person?" The answer to major life questions may be elusive, but a woman *can* judge her "performance" as a woman today by measuring pounds, calories, hours of exercise and clothing size.

Like Jennifer, some adult women slip over the edge into eating disorders and severe body image despair. Adult women and adolescents with eating disorder share some characteristics, like using body obsession to cope with developmental challenges and identity development. They share the tendency to translate difficult feelings into the language of fat, and play out their distress on the canvas of the body. Likewise, younger and older women live together in a culture rife with body myths that are toxic for women's body image and self-worth.

However, there are significant differences between the two populations. Grown women feel that they should know better than to have such teenage problems. They tend to have more embarrassment and shame about body disturbances, feeling that this distress is less legitimate and not a worthwhile reason to seek help. Adult women also have more serious everyday responsibilities; consequently, they have more people to disappoint if they fail. For all these reasons, it feels much harder to commit time and energy to address eating and body image disorders.

> Perfectionism is not a quest for the best. It is a pursuit of the worst in ourselves, the part that tells us that nothing we do will ever be good enough—that we should try harder.[3]
>
> Julia Cameron

Jennifer's story is not unique. Millions of adult women in the United States struggle with weight obsession and body image dissatisfaction—committing enormous time and energy to restricting their food intake.

Most of this dieting is the yo-yo variety. Lost weight is regained, often with additional pounds, due to the metabolic chaos caused by repetitive restriction cycles—which trigger still more rounds of dieting. Weight cycling can actually increase the risk for health problems and premature death.[4] The yo-yo label aptly describes how often women's lives and sense of well-being spin up and down with the success or failure of their diets.

Women today inherit a multigenerational fixation with appearance and shape. For example, a 1983 *Glamour* magazine survey of 33,000 readers showed that 75 percent thought they were overweight, while only 25 percent of them actually were overweight. In other words, *half* of the survey respondents had severely distorted images of their own bodies. Meanwhile, 42 percent of readers said losing weight would make them the happiest—twice the percentage of those who chose work success or dating a man they admired.[5]

Decades later, our current generation of women is still saddled with distorted body image and body dissatisfaction.

A 2012 study found that eating disorder symptoms, dieting and body checking behaviors, and weight and shape concerns are still widely endorsed by women over 50.[6] Among these more mature women, researchers found:

* 79 percent report that weight/shape affects their self–image
* 41 percent weigh themselves daily
* 60 percent report that their concerns about weight and shape negatively affect their lives
* 13.3 percent report current eating disorder symptoms
* 8 percent report purging.

The news is no better for adult women under 50. A 2008 study of US women aged 25–45[7] found:

- 67 percent (excluding those with diagnosed eating disorders) are trying to lose weight
- 53 percent of current dieters are already at a healthy weight
- 39 percent say concerns about weight or eating interfere with their happiness
- 37 percent regularly skip meals to lose weight
- 27 percent would be upset if they gained five pounds
- 26 percent cut out whole food groups
- 16 percent have dieted on less than 1,000 calories a day
- 13 percent smoke to lose weight
- 12 percent often eat when they are not hungry; 49 percent sometimes do
- 75 percent report eating behaviors or symptoms consistent with eating disorders.

Even women over 60 battle the Perfect Problem. A 2006 study of Austrian women aged 60–70[8] found that:

- 80 percent "controlled their weight"
- 60 percent reported body dissatisfaction, regardless of their weight or Body Mass Index (BMI)
- 4 percent met the criteria for clinical eating disorders
- another 4 percent met criteria for subclinical eating disorders.

Clearly, the passage of time isn't helping aging women feel more at peace with their bodies—or making things better for younger women following them into adulthood. The legacy of body image and weight obsession is passed down from one generation to the next, reinforced for women of all ages by the body myths of our youth- and appearance-oriented culture.

These figures illustrate how many North American women live in the prison of perfectionism, searching for self-worth (and worth to others) in the mirror, in the size on our clothing, and in the number on the scale. This perfect problem promotes the myth that we can find life's meaning and the answer to every challenge in the shape of our bodies.

Perfect Myths

Myths are stories that help us make sense of our lives and of life itself. Myths grow from, and are bound to, the culture of the family and/or the culture of the larger society. They are not inherently bad things (think Santa Claus!).

Myths help us make sense of life, and hold off feelings of anxiety, but that doesn't make every myth good for us. Deeply rooted in culture, myths tend to reinforce our perceptions of reality, but not to question those perceptions. Myths about women's bodies are deeply embedded in our psyches, too. The pursuit of today's impossible standards for women reinforces a false "reality" which says: "Changing my body equals changing my life and brings me closer to perfection."

> Worship your own body and beauty and sexual allure and you will always feel ugly, and when time and age start showing, you will die a million deaths before they finally plant you. If they are where you tap real meaning in life — then you will never have enough.[9]
>
> David Foster Wallace

Living in body myths, our desire to change our shape overwhelms the desire to *be in* our body. Paradoxically, being "on a diet" seems intrinsically healthy and good—something to be admired and imitated. We perceive women in Weight Watchers®, Jenny Craig® or Ideal Protein as dedicated, committed and good. So why give up dieting?

Unfortunately, body myths obscure important facts. The most common yo-yo diets undermine nutrition and well-being. They increase the risks for cardiovascular disease, type II diabetes, osteoporosis, eating disorders and some cancers (see Chapter 2). Research finds women who are depressed engage in more unhealthy dieting behaviors than women with fewer depressive symptoms —a sign that they may obsess about body image in a futile effort to feed or soothe much deeper hungers.[10] They may be attempting to change how their bodies look rather than making peace with the inevitable, natural and sometimes painful changes of aging—and the rapid evolution of women's roles.

Living as Immigrants

> The state of a woman's health is indeed completely tied up with the culture in which she lives and her position within it.[11]
>
> Christiane Northrup

Our lives—and the ongoing importance of our bodies' appearance in our lives—are substantially different than they were for our grandmothers (and, possibly, our mothers) at our age. The opportunities open to us are considerably wider than before, and the expectations are much higher. The meaning of success and "good enough" are light years beyond our foremothers' definition.

It's as if women have immigrated to a new world. Most mature women started their journey through adolescence expecting to arrive in a women's world similar to the one their mothers inhabited. But today's world has dramatically different expectations for women than a generation ago.

In a sense, we are suffering culture shock. In the past 50 years, the modern world of womanhood has changed radically, in visible and invisible ways. Our foremothers often can't guide us through this new territory, and no Google Map can help us find a safe route through the pitfalls of "perfect" expectations.

Like newly arrived immigrants, many of us aren't prepared for the new cultural mores, and can't quite grasp the requirements and demands. We are pioneers with few role models or guides for navigating this transformed and novel culture of womanhood, with its new stressors, opportunities, freedoms and advantages.

Like geographical culture shock, this transition is emotionally trying and confusing. Among other challenges, we experience cognitive dissonance between what our female ancestors expected of themselves (and what we grew up expecting to expect of *our*selves) and what modern culture expects of women.

Feeling uprooted from the world of our foremothers, we crave familiarity and security. In response, many of us grab for our culture's chimerical "beauty" standard as the way to acculturate ourselves and organize our lives. Rather than unlocking all the potential in this new land of opportunity, as successful immigrants do, the perfect problem convinces us to measure our success by how strictly we manage our bodies.

Keeping Herself Up

As we grow up, we form our identity, at least in part, by defining ourselves in opposition to someone or something else. Since young girls identify strongly with their mothers, we also feel some pressure to differentiate ourselves from mom to become separate (eventually adult) people. For women born after 1950, this differentiation often centers on the body because the ways our mothers or grandmothers looked and aged isn't good enough for today's standards of perfection.

We don't dare to "let ourselves go," as women did in the past. We are today's women, and are supposed to be in control of everything—including signs that the aging process is taking its natural course. We feel failure if we detect Mom or Grandma when we look in the mirror.

As our grandmothers aged, they still cared about appearance and often criticized a woman for not keeping herself up. But such criticism was likely to be aimed at a contemporary with questionable taste in make-up or a colorblind fashion sense. When it came to body shape, the parameters were pretty broad.

Today, we criticize an adult woman because she no longer has the body of a 16- or 20-year old. Although natural for the adult female body, all weight gain is considered wrong. We scrutinize any gray hair, any wrinkle, any sign of natural aging—in others and ourselves.

> And so, to be fat is to deal with people's projections that you are a loser, whether you feel like one or not; and, to be thin is to live in fear of exposure of your inner loser-ness. Clearly, changing one's body size provides no solution to the existential question of how to claim one's imperfection as a human being.[12]
>
> Deb Burgard

Our grandmothers had few medical technologies at their disposal to help manage their bodies. While they wore girdles and make-up, we spend hours and dollars undergoing cosmetic surgery, experimenting with the latest diets or weight loss products, and hiring trainers to sculpt our physique. We have manicures, pedicures, false nails and eyelashes. We wax hair off our eyebrows, legs and "bikini line;" go "tanning;" or use chemicals to look bronzed. Collectively, US women will spend $62.46 Billion on cosmetics during 2016[13]—at least 12.5 times more than political action committees and two dozen candidates will spend on the 2016 Presidential election.[14]

Another huge, but seldom discussed difference between the generations is how much more visible modern women's bodies are in public. Most of us are more active in careers and public life than previous generations. Always on display, we are endlessly criticized for transgressing that ever-shifting fine line between being too sexy or not sexy enough. Meanwhile, sexualized images of female bodies saturate everyday media, fueling body myths and distorting our idea of the ideal female form. We have no access to the body image sanctuaries our grandmothers did.

We have emigrated to an appearance-obsessed culture, where it is considered normal to work out our insecurities in and on our body image—how we think we look. We struggle to live up to (and make sense of) bizarre cultural norms like: "What you see is what you get" or "You can never be too rich or too thin."

The Shape of History

Let's be clear: the body is essential to identity, because we couldn't be alive (and hence have an identity) without it.

For millennia, humans have pondered the relationship between mind and body, flesh and spirit, psychology and physiology, or body and soul. One of the very few areas approaching consensus across the history of spiritual, philosophical, medical, psychological and religious thought is this: the body is not the sole source of our identity and purpose. For example, Judeo-Christian tradition calls the body a temple which we should keep open and healthy to help our souls flourish, and thus be helpful to others.

Many spiritual writers think metaphorically about the body as a vessel or tool that holds, nourishes and conveys our essence (or whatever other spiritual metaphor best helps us understand the spark of life).

The body gives us the apparatus to think, speak, touch, feel, listen, taste, smell and sense ourselves and what is around us. It provides the means to express our self and shape our relationships with our self and those we love. We are in the body when we reflect on life's ongoing difficulties and joys, and when we grow in response to them.

But *we are not our bodies*. You are not your body. Your body is only the vehicle; it is not the journey or the destination.

Even in the most woman-friendly culture we could imagine, the body—and our relationship with it—would be only *a part* of how we experience and respond to life transitions. Unfortunately, our culture is not so woman-friendly. Its distorted perspective presents our bodies as the principal (and sometimes only) canvas on which we paint our future.

The Shape of Adulthood

Remember the intense concern about how we looked when we were teenagers? Popularity seemed to depend on who was "cutest" and had the coolest clothes. This competition for acceptance fed on and intensified the insecurity of adolescence, the essential transition from a childhood identity to an adult one.

Identity is central to a person's sense of self. Our identity integrates different parts of ourselves (for example: daughter, sister, student, friend, mother, childless, single, girlfriend, volunteer, employee, Iranian Sunni, Irish Catholic, or Russian Jew) into a cohesive whole. Ideally, a self-perception feels firm and stable.

But identity is also multidimensional and continues to develop throughout life. For instance, you may be single, then married, and then divorced. This fluid, lifelong identity process builds on a foundation constructed from:

- family dynamics
- early experiences
- ethnic, socio-economic and cultural background
- religious training and beliefs
- emotional and mental capacities
- gender identity
- sexual orientation
- temperament and personality
- physical attributes
- body image (especially for Western females).

Adolescence and childhood are *not* the only identity development periods in our lives. Adulthood is also filled with change, by turns dramatic, subtle and mundane. A modern women's development isn't anywhere close to being over when she becomes a legal adult at age 18 or 21. A woman traveling through adulthood deals with ongoing developmental issues (an aging body, mothering, mortality, empty nesting and more), which can be tougher than her adolescent challenges.

However, many adult transitions lack the rituals that mark and signal moments of childhood (our first steps or first day of school) and adolescence (our first bra or first period). There are few grown-up equivalents of confirmation ceremonies, proms, or graduation parties to help us remember, recognize and celebrate the transitions between one phase of life and the next.

It may seem odd to think that adults have developmental issues. But while adolescence requires that we synthesize our childhood self with the new demands of puberty and future adulthood, adult development also requires synthesis of past and emerging identities. Even from the earliest years of adulthood, we move from one role to the next—frequently maintaining multiple roles at the same time. We experience regular transitions: first full-time job, first time living on our own, serious relationships with significant others, marriage and leaving the people and places of our youth. Our roles in relation to our parents may change from being the "child" to mutual friend, to caretaker as they age. Adulthood also brings significant bodily transitions due to pregnancy, menopause and the aging process.

At our adult crossroads, we may feel unsure of ourselves when old beliefs and assumptions are severely tested or rendered obsolete. We may choose new paths, reorganize how we think, and change how we live in relationships. These transitions can affect our personality and bring major shifts in social roles—what our family, community and culture expect from us.

Our adult responsibilities (managing jobs, family, money, community, etc.) leave little time to pay attention to what is happening inside us, let alone to reflect on the impact of all these events and transitions.

Nevertheless, the impact remains. Essential questions stir inside, as we grow further away from our youth and closer to old age and, ultimately, death. In *Passages: Predictable Crises of Adult Life*,[15] Gail Sheehy describes the sensation of moving through the midpoint of our lives: "Deep down a change begins to register in those gut-level perceptions of safety and danger, time and no-time, aliveness and stagnation, self and others."

A sense of "deadline" springs from our ticking biological clock. If we are childless, we may feel growing urgency to get pregnant. If we are already mothers, we may sense career paths closing down. If we juggle both nurturing and career, the "what-about-me?" alarm may sound. Because family nurture still falls primarily to women, men are less like to feel the same sort of crisis. Thus, our "deadline" concerns may put us out of sync with our partner, a problem in its own right.

Adult transitions do share one quality with childhood transitions: they seldom happen with a snap of the fingers. Major changes are likely to turn our own world a bit topsy-turvy. New perspectives may be valuable, but we sometimes lack the internal mechanisms or social support to meet these challenges easily. Shaking up our sense of identity can bring unsettling feelings. Pile these challenges atop our experience of being immigrants in modern culture, and it's no wonder women struggle to keep a cohesive sense of self.

Shaping Adult Development

Naomi, a New York public relations executive, was 45 when she began compulsive dieting and addictive use of laxatives to control her weight. Soon, things spun out of control. Naomi had full-blown bulimia and carried just over 100 pounds on her five-foot nine-inch frame. She told the *New York Times*:

> My whole life was shaped by this. I didn't want to take trips with people or visit my in-laws because they had only one bathroom. I couldn't control my husband's drinking, and I didn't feel as though I could control anything.[16]

Naomi was looking for a way to control the profound challenges and changes facing her. Desperate to gain a hold on some part of her life, she turned to controlling her weight. Bingeing and purging became a pernicious self-soothing strategy.

Eventually Naomi began to realize the risks of what she was doing. She became desperate to avoid a heart attack or other life-threatening illness. But it took six scary years of suffering before she finally sought therapy. She began to see how the natural stresses and losses of midlife conspired with our cultures notions of beauty to plummet her into the deadly cycle of eating disorders.

Like Naomi, many women use their bodies to answer the difficult questions of womanhood such as these:

- What is feminine?
- What is adult?
- What kind of woman am I?
- Am I good enough?
- Who am I as a female in this culture and in this body?
- Am I living up to the standard I'm supposed to?
- What example of womanliness am I setting for my children?

Because our world is fast-paced, and driven by performance and image, we have few opportunities to explore such open-ended questions.

The answers are not always obvious and the solutions not easy to grasp. But we know our body is here, no matter what else happens. And so, baffled or frustrated by life's hazy transitions, we often seize our body as an obvious and concrete thing to shape, force to behave, manipulate and "figure out." In a sense, we use (or misuse) our body's outside shape to process or silence the feelings, doubt, indecision and insecurity that adult development stirs inside us.

Meanwhile, our culture consistently values women for our bodies. So it is not unusual for us to judge ourselves by how well we "control" our bodies, especially when everything else (including, sometimes, our bodies themselves) feel out of control. We are uncertain whether we are up to life's tasks, but if we can shape the "right" body or appearance, we believe that we can feel (or at least look) like we have control. That's the perfect problem—the circular and never-ending search to be "good enough" women. We battle our bodies instead of finally accepting them, loving them, and being grateful for all they allow us to do.

Step Back Exercise I

Do this alone, with a friend or in a small group of women you trust. Take time to talk about your feelings and insights afterwards.

- Stand comfortably, preferably without shoes so you can feel the ground or floor, with enough space that you can move backward and forward several feet. Close your eyes and relax.
- Take one step back and imagine that you are stepping into your mother's body when she was the same age you are now. Take a few minutes to get used to being in her body and mind.
- Take another step backward and step into the body of your mother's mother. Again take time to get used to being in your grandmother's life and in her body. (If didn't know your mother, grandmother, or great-grandmother, imagine living during her time in history.)
- Next, step into your great grandmother's body and let yourself experience what her life and her experience of her body was like.
- As your great grandmother, ask yourself these questions:
  - What are my major concerns or worries in life?
  - What are my primary sources of satisfaction? Of comfort?
  - What is my position in my society: what are its limitations, opportunities, privileges, responsibilities?
  - How do I feel about my body? How important is it to my sense of self?
  - What are my worries about my health? About my body?

- – What pressures do I feel to prove myself?
- – Do I feel I must be perfect to survive or succeed?
- – What do I feel I must be to survive or succeed?

- Take a few minutes to absorb these insights and then step forward to being your grandmother. Ask yourself the same questions. Again take some time to absorb this experience.
- Then step forward to being your mother and ask the same questions once more. Again take some time to absorb this experience.
- Now step forward to being yourself and ask the same questions once more. What are the common threads in these experiences? What are the differences? How did body or beauty concerns evolve throughout these generations? Where and when did the perfect problem appear in these stories? What do you feel about this experience? In what ways do you feel connected to the past? In what ways do you feel alone, disconnected, like an emotional and cultural immigrant? What surprised you as you traversed these bodies and generations?

Talk about your feelings and insights with friends. Take some time to write these perceptions down in a journal so you can reflect on them over time.

Notes

1 Mount Holyoke College Commencement Address, May 23, 1999. See www.mtholyoke.edu/offices/comm/csj/990604/Quindlen.html 13 (retrieved August 12, 2015).
2 *Body Thieves: Help Girls Reclaim Their Natural Bodies and Become Physically Active* (Vancouver, BC: Sala Books, 2002) p. 21.
3 *The Artist's Way: A Spiritual Path to Higher Creativity* (New York: Putnam, 2002) p. 120.
4 Linda Bacon and Lucy Aphramor (2011) "Weight Science: Evaluating the evidence for a paradigm shift." *Nutrition Journal*, 10 (9), 1–13.
5 "Feeling fat in a thin society." *Glamour*, February 1984, 198–201 and 251–252.
6 Danielle A. Gagne, Ann Von Holle, Kimberly A. Brownley, Cristin D. Runfola, Sara Hofmeier, Kateland E. Branch and Cynthia M. Bulik (2012) "Eating disorder symptoms and weight and shape concerns in a large web-based convenience sample of women ages 50 and above: Results of the gender and body image (GABI) study." *International Journal of Eating Disorders*, 45 (7), 832–844.
7 Lauren Reba-Harrelson, Ann Von Holle, Robert M. Hamer, Rebecca Swann, Mae Lynn Reyes and Cynthia M. Bulik (2009) "Patterns and prevalence of disordered eating and weight control behaviors in women ages 25–45." *Eating and Weight Disorders*, 14 (4), 190–198.
8 Barbara Mangweth-Matzek, Claudia Ines Rupp, Armand Hausmann, Karin Assmayr, Edith Mariacher, Georg Kemmler, Alexandra B. Whitworth

and Wilfried Biebl (2006) "Never too old for eating disorders or body dissatisfaction: A community study of elderly women." *International Journal of Eating Disorders*, 39 (7), 583–586.

9 *This Is Water: Some Thoughts, Delivered on a Significant Occasion, about Living a Compassionate Life* (New York: Little Brown, 2009) p. 101.

10 Meghan M. Gillen, Charlotte N. Markey and Patrick M. Markey (2012) "An examination of dieting behaviors among adults: Links with depression." *Eating Behaviors*, 13 (2), 88–93.

11 *Women's Bodies, Women's Wisdom: Creating Physical and Emotional Health and Healing* (New York: Bantam Dell, 2006) p. xxxiv.

12 "What's weight got to do with it? Weight neutrality in the health at every size paradigm and its implications for clinical practice." In Margo Maine, Beth Hartman McGilley and Douglas Bunnell (Eds.) *Treatment of Eating Disorders: Bridging the Research-Practice Gap* (London: Elsevier, 2010) p. 23.

13 Statista.com, "Revenue of the cosmetic industry in the United States from 2002 to 2016 (in billion US dollars)." See http://www.statista.com/statistics/243742/revenue-of-the-cosmetic-industry-in-the-us/ (retrieved August 10, 2015).

14 *The Hill*, "The $5 billion presidential campaign?" January 21, 2015. See http://thehill.com/blogs/ballot-box/presidential-races/230318-the-5-billion-campaign (retrieved August 10, 2015). $62.46 billion (see previous note) divided by $5 billion equals 12.49.

15 New York: Bantam, 1984, p. 242.

16 Ginia Bellafant, "When midlife seems just an empty plate. "*The New York Times*, March 9, 2003. See http://www.nytimes.com/2003/03/09/style/when-midlife-seems-just-an-empty-plate.html (retrieved August 10, 2015).

2   Women's Bodies, Women's Lives

What baby ever wished
that his mother was slimmer,
her hips narrower,
her breasts less full?[1]

Sydney Smith

So what is the actual state of our psychological, spiritual, emotional, relational and physical lives as adult women? Does it continue to be a state of regular change, growth, loss and transition? The development of our identity doesn't stop just because we've passed through the gates of childhood and adolescence.

As they did in our early years, transitions bring growth, and require us to leave something behind. As toddlers, we left the security of being always held and coddled. But in exchange, we began experiencing the world in independent and exciting ways. The first time we rode a bike without training wheels, we felt simultaneously scared of falling and liberated by our new ability to explore the neighborhood more widely and autonomously. The fear is real, but so is the reward of facing the fear and working through it.

This chapter describes transitions common to adult women's lives, and examines how they influence our body image, sense of self and the ways we respond by trying to craft a "perfect" image. We'll explore women's bodies, work, families and relationships.

Women's Bodies

Pregnancy and Childbirth

Women's ability to bear children allows our species to continue. So, we might expect that every aspect of our bodies would be widely and enthusiastically celebrated—including how pregnancy and childbirth change our bodies.

Instead, our perfect-appearance-obsessed culture is far more enamored with a woman whose appearance generates male sexual feelings and/or looks like she's "easy." Visibly pregnant models aren't centerfold models and Madonna's revealing outfits get more media attention than a nation of madonnas bearing children.

Some of my clients agonize over pregnancy weight gain and contemplate having their tubes tied to prevent natural reshaping. For others, pregnancy is the one time they feel free to eat and to actually enjoy a fuller, feminine shape and appetite, while appreciating the wonderful things their bodies can do naturally.

During her teens and 20s, Meredith's life was shot through with painful symptoms of anorexia. Marriage and pregnancy seemed to calm those demons. But Meredith also found herself craving the endless hours she once spent shopping, dieting and tanning with friends and the flirtatious spontaneity of life before marriage and motherhood. So Meredith resumed her dangerous anorexic behaviors as she tried to connect to that "carefree" life through a slimmer body that (she hoped) betrayed no sign that she was now a mother.

Pregnancy and childbirth literature reflect this ambiguity (at best) and distress (at worst) with advice on restoring buff abs and butt, so no one can tell you were ever pregnant. Supermarket tabloids, magazines and social networking sites flaunt images of celebrities who gain little during pregnancy and then instantly return to their "original" weight (with the help of nannies, personal trainers, chefs and perhaps an eating disorder). In its ongoing obsession with women's bodies, the media even coined the word "pregorexia."

However, nature designed women's bodies to be different after childbirth, so that we can nurse our children, carry them around, and more easily give birth to subsequent children. The adult female body also starts preparing for menopause well before its onset. Attempts to reverse or deny that process only dissipate our energy and open us up to dangerous physical and emotional problems.

Fertility and Infertility

Fertility problems are hard to discuss openly or socially. Women struggling with infertility may feel desperately inadequate because they can't fulfill this "key part" of being a woman. They may also believe that fertility problems disappoint spouses, parents and in-laws—a dynamic that often drives strong feelings of guilt and depression underground.

Modern medical efforts to overcome infertility may traumatize a woman's relationship to her body, as she focuses intently on ovulation, temperature and other body functions. Invasive fertility work-ups create physical and emotional stress directly tied to her body. While interacting with health care professionals, she may feel de-womanized and dehumanized, on top of feeling that her body is failing.

Meanwhile, fertility treatments and drugs tend to increase weight and water retention. A woman undergoing these treatments may feel out of control and hyper-critical of her highly scrutinized body, as well as deeply disappointed with its (her) performance. As she goes through the hit-and-miss fertility process, she may be on a roller coaster of high hopes followed by smashed dreams.

As sexual intercourse is analyzed and programmed to promote conception, intimate relationships can also swell with tension that threatens natural spontaneity and sexual pleasure. A woman may become very critical of her sexual relationships, and therefore, of her body's role in sex and conception.

If a woman had an eating disorder earlier in life, she may also feel guilty that the disorder caused or contributed to her infertility. Although there is no evidence that infertility causes eating disorders, the body-centered strain and tension of overcoming infertility might prompt women to develop (or return to) disordered eating rituals or exercise abuse to self-soothe. A number of my patients had severe disordered eating and body image despair sparked by reactions to their infertility treatments.

Menopause

Ann was in her late 50s and married 35 years before she sought help for her recent onset of bulimia. A successful business woman with three adult children and a grandchild, Ann had navigated many twists and turns in life. Before menopause, she was weight conscious, but not pathologically so.

After menopause, however, Ann gained a few pounds that she could not seem to shed. "My old tricks didn't work anymore," she said. "I made a conscious, intellectual decision to start making myself vomit. I had seen many magazine articles about purging and watched made-for-TV movies about bulimia. I saw vomiting as an acceptable option, on the same level as Weight Watchers or the Atkins diet."

When I described the health risks of bulimia for a woman her age, Ann was deeply affected and felt motivated to change her behavior. Because Ann's bulimia was not yet deeply embedded in her identity, these changes were easier than for many other patients. She stopped vomiting and began to address the problems that seemed to underlie her bulimia.

Even with a stable marriage and family, friends, financial resources and a strong business reputation, Ann still felt afraid of menopause, becoming a grandmother and life in retirement without the daily feedback that her career provided. She felt lingering grief over the death of her parents, the loss of her own youth and the loss of "control" over her weight.

Why would menopause bring on a violent case of bulimia for a successful and well-supported woman who tolerated significant life transitions in the past? Menopause brings unruly hot flashes, slowing metabolism, vaginal dryness and the other physical changes despised by our youth-focused culture. We feel ambushed by weight gain, hormonal mood swings and the "imperfection" of ageing.

Few women have debilitating menopausal symptoms, but nowadays *any* symptom of this natural process seems to justify medical and pharmaceutical intervention. We think we need to medically manage menopause–which previous generations of women had little or no call to do. Then, if medically marketed strategies trump nature's time-tested menopausal methods, and we still don't have girlish bodies, we may feel stupid and inadequate.

Our grandmothers didn't pathologize menopause; it was usually a relatively unremarkable feature of their busy lives. For centuries, rich cultural rituals marked both menarche (a girl's first period) and menopause. For example, in many historic cultures, women used a "Red Tent" to mark major life transitions together.[2] When a woman reached menopause, she was inducted into the corps of wise older women (known as crones) responsible for the tent.

In our culture, rituals of honoring aging women have been swapped for rituals of hormone replacement therapy. This attitude undermines the pride of reaching new levels of wisdom or of our release from the monthly "visit" of menstruation. Sadly, it also mirrors what happens to our daughters and granddaughters.

Before they start menstruating, girls in our culture tend to be strong, outspoken and bold. But as they enter adolescence, girls tend to lose that confidence, taking their feelings and insight underground, lest they upset someone else. The pioneering research of Dr. Carol Gilligan, Dr. Lyn Mikel Brown, and others describes this as "the silencing of girls' voices."[3] Many of us struggle throughout adulthood to regain some of that voice and the potency we felt as sassy 10-year-olds.

> There is no greater power in the world today than the zest of a post-menopausal woman.[4]
>
> Margaret Mead

I imagine menopause as a liberating transition to recapturing the enthusiasm and clarity of young girls. We can seize permission to shed the weight of sexual expectations and reproductive pressures, entering a period of "peaceful potency" when women become less inhibited, more confident and more action-oriented.[5] Writer Betty Friedan calls aging an opportunity for *both* sexes "to become more and more themselves."[6] Can we view this phase of life as an adventure and evolution (e.g., Carly Fiorina running to become President at age 62 and Hilary Clinton at age 69[7]), rather than a dead end?

Instead of adopting a zesty outlook, however, many of us still go to war with our bodies during and after menopause. In Pursuit of Perfection, we critique our bodies, dwelling on their failure to measure up against consumer images of beauty.

From Intrusion to Invisibility

Our culture's obsession with looking young does not spring from a biological necessity or immutable natural force. Many other cultures respect and emulate older people as fonts of wisdom and cultural continuity. US women traveling in Europe are often surprised that men find them attractive even if they *look their age*.

Meanwhile back home, we may feel ambivalent when intrusive, objectifying and threatening male comments about our bodies become less frequent (or stop altogether). Germaine Greer describes how this "loss" of random leering commentary means a loss of personal status:

> Though [the] excessive visibility [of her youth] was anguish, her present invisibility is disorienting. She had not realized how much she depended upon her physical presence, at shop counters, at the garage, on the bus. For the first time in her life she finds she has to raise her voice or wait endlessly while other people push in front of her.[8]

My first "I'm invisible!" experience happened when (in my 40s) I reached the front of the line at a local bagel shop. The 30-something man behind the counter looked right past me, started chatting with a 20-something police officer behind me—taking his order before mine. I was angry and shocked that my simple right to be served suddenly disappeared, along with the assumption that my physical presence automatically mattered. My most basic prerogatives felt abruptly stripped away.

I also was stunned by the revulsion toward getting older that rose up *within me*. Long-held feelings of honor and respect for older women's wisdom crashed into my sudden, passionate resistance to being seen (or, more accurately, being ignored) as old.

Many of us resist "invisibility" by dieting, coloring our hair, having cosmetic surgery, exercising and staying tanned in order to look young and noticeable—even if it prolongs male leering.

Of course, as we traverse womanhood, the body is less "forgiving" than it used to be. We can't get into yoga poses as gracefully and easily as we could at 20 or 30 (and my days of eight minute miles are long gone). The arm I broke during a half-marathon at age 64 required months of immobilization, humbling and unfamiliar dependence on others and intense physical therapy. In other words, the body is a concrete reminder of that essential reality: we and our beautifully imperfect bodies are getting—like everyone else's.

Death

All humans have death and birth in common. The death of a peer when we are young seems to defy the natural order of things. But as we age, illness and death become part of our landscape. We start noticing the ages of people in the obituaries, even if they are strangers.

Human beings respond to death in the context of our feelings about previous losses. At the same time, each new death has unique impact and symbolism. For example, my father died when I was 20. More than 30 years later, my mother's death made my goodbye to my dad feel much more final.

A parent's death brings profound, transformative and often frightening shifts in our identity.

- I must act grown up now, because no one is there to rescue me anymore.
- I'm the one responsible.
- I am now a matriarch at the vanguard of my family.

A mother's death can bring particular identity challenges. As girls, we identify closely with Mom. Then, adolescence and other developmental imperatives lead many of us away emotionally, defining ourselves by the ways we are different from Mom. Many daughters and mothers eventually reconnect as adults, sharing the experience of being a partner, mother and other adult roles.

For most of my life, I felt close to my mother *and* saw myself as very different from her. My need to focus on all our differences diminished during my mother's final years. Instead, I began to search for and cherish our similarities, including physical ones. I saw my mother as a natural beauty with no frills; and I felt drawn to that same style.

When she fell ill late in life, I took over the "mothering" role to care for her. This natural experience brought us a level of peace and intimacy that was both joyful and painful—a truly mixed blessing which helps me feel good about her ongoing presence and influence in my life.

As a mother ages, her daughter's desire to find and touch the common ground can bring new levels of self-discovery. But this may be difficult if you haven't had the opportunity to arrive at a healthy adult relationship with your mother. In many unconscious ways, the legacy of her relationship to food, body and pursuit of perfection shapes your own.

For example, Catherine's mother died suddenly before they'd yet entered a more adult phase in their relationship. For several years, Catherine felt she had nothing to hang onto after Mom's death. She used a chaotic relationship with food to act out her confusion about her mom, her grief and her deep disconnection. Depressed and full of regret over lost opportunities, her discomfort with her weight and body image erupted into bulimia.

When she finally entered treatment, Catherine recalled how frequently mom dieted, controlled her eating in front of others, and used food to soothe herself when she was alone and depressed. While no longer able to ask mom about these issues, Catherine still found ways to identify and connect spiritually to her mother. Eventually, she gave up her symptoms of restricting, bingeing and purging—and discovered greater peace with her body and with food.

Death reminds us that time is limited. We may reexamine what we're doing with our life; take inventory of whether we've done "enough" and ask ourselves questions such as:

- What is the meaning of my life?
- Should I quit my job and enjoy retirement or the different challenges of a new career?
- Or should I stay where I am and accomplish more here?
- Should I stay in this relationship?

Surviving the death of a loved one can get us thinking seriously, or even compulsively, about the threat of illness. In an effort to prevent disease, we may develop heightened concern or phobic obsession about food, weight, body and exercise.

Our culture's obsession with youthfulness stems in part from a deep-seated resistance to the very idea of death. Many other cultures tend to be more open about death and its impact, taking this natural phenomenon more in stride. On the other hand, our culture has a "denial of death" which both reinforces and feeds on our over-glorification of youth.[9]

This pervasive denial becomes a huge barrier when one of our loved ones dies. We are allowed very little permission to mourn and openly acknowledge a death.

The pressure to deny grief can be particularly hard on women, because we are acculturated to live up to the expectations and demands of others. Yet, we are also acculturated to be closely connected to others, making a loved one's loss especially hard. If others are expecting us to "move on" after a major loss like death, it's easy to feel that our grief isn't valuable— or even that it isn't real.

Miscarriage or Death of a Child

Miscarriage and infant death are particularly disenfranchised, private and isolating losses; often minimized by people around us—including our families. A lack of support suggests to us that grieving an infant death or miscarriage isn't important or worth the effort. This creates inner conflict and turmoil, because the child is very real to the parents, whether or not the child was actually born.

A miscarriage or infant death may lead us to castigate ourselves and our bodies with questions like "Why couldn't I do more?" These reactions are normal, and ultimately pass if we are allowed to grieve. But they may also lead to severe self-criticism of the body, opening the door to physical and psychological self-flagellation, such as disordered eating.

Some forms of death, like suicides and drug overdoses, are especially stigmatized, with surviving loved ones getting even less support than the pittance allotted for "more acceptable" deaths. Once again, guilty thoughts like "How did I fail him?" complicate the grieving process, despite mounds of evidence showing, for example, that depression and addiction are real diseases.

Conflict also springs from the different ways individuals mourn. Under the stress of a child's death, one parent may grow impatient with how the other one grieves, or else both may learn new ways to support one another. As a father wrote after he and his wife lost their baby: "A miscarriage will either pull you together or pull you apart."

Surviving a loss is simply very stressful and sad. Our grief is complicated by how firmly Western culture denies death and delegitimizes grief. Periods of bingeing and/or appetite loss are not uncommon during early stages of mourning, as we shape and soothe the sadness. However, continuing these patterns is dangerous, especially for women with a history of body image despair and eating disorders. Instead of trying to resolve our grief by manipulating our bodies, we must embrace it in the company of genuine fellow humans—even if this means defying cultural conventions about death, grief and the value of life.

Women's Work

> The ability to take pride in your own work is one of the hallmarks of sanity. Take away the ability to both work and be proud of it and you can drive anyone insane.[10]
>
> Nikki Giovanni

At Work and At Home

Women with eating and body image concerns are likely to be talented, resourceful and accomplished—but seldom see themselves that way. Many other women also toil to value their professional worth.

How often have we buried our many achievements under a mound of regret over one failure? What criteria do we use to evaluate our career accomplishments and ourselves? Men struggle with these questions too, but a man's success criteria tend to be simpler (and simplistic): do career, and measure success by salary growth and occupational advancement.

As contemporary women, we feel like we must master money and career—along with child-rearing, family logistics and the emotional life of relationships. And we have to do it all perfectly. If our career feels under control (or, God forbid, prospers), we feel guilty about shortchanging our family. If we devote attention to family matters, we worry that our career advancement and sense of accomplishment will suffer.

According to a 2013 Pew Research Center survey, women were three times more likely than men to say that being a working parent limits their career advancement. Women more frequently reduced their hours or even terminated employment to take care of their children.[11] Women and men both tend to think of fathers as second-class parents, giving them a pass on child-rearing responsibilities—and child-rearing joys, too. Couples who choose "alternative" ways of balancing family and work generally get little support.

Expectations of perfection are palpable for women—as is the disappointing feeling that we haven't mastered every responsibility and opportunity that comes our way. Too often we blame and shame ourselves for workplace sexual harassment and gender pay inequities—rather than seeing these problems as systemic cultural failures.

In addition, a "highly attractive" appearance is considered essential for women's success, even in the most conventional professions. Read about the murky path one woman realtor must constantly tread:

> My clothes, my make-up, my weight—they are all an ordeal every day. If I look "too good," people either don't take me seriously, or accuse me of being seductive and manipulative to make a sale. That attitude is especially strong among many of my male colleagues. On the other hand, looking "too plain" projects an unprofessional image. How can I make it to "in between" every day? I can't even tell for sure what "in-between" is! An outfit that seems to work well most days will unexpectedly strike a colleague or customer as too sexy or too frumpy on other days. I feel like my body and clothes are on display as much as they are for any supermodel. But if I was a model, at least I'd know what I was supposed to look like. When it comes to my "professional look," most days I feel like I don't know and I can't win.[12]

If we worry that we are dedicating too much to our career, or pursuing (and achieving) a "too male" career path, we may feel the need to compensate, developing appearance, weight, or eating problems in order to balance what's perceived as "masculine" behavior. We may be tempted to act girlish and flirty to offset assertive or aggressive work behaviors that might be seen as offensive.

Many people still see jobs as optional for women. But most women work to support our families, whether in tandem with a partner or alone as a single parent. News stories about women abandoning the career track make it hard not to feel guilty or ask, "Why can't I do what my kids need me to do, and give all my time to them?"

Decisions about balancing family and work are seldom easy or simple. This ambiguity sometimes reinforces our desire to seek more measurable answers by working to perfect our body, the one element we've been told (mistakenly) that we can master.

Can we find ways to challenge these perfectly unrealistic expectations—making choices that fit us, our needs, and (most of the time) also fit our family's needs?

Competing with Younger Women

Women of all ages are more visible than ever in the workplace. Previous generations of women worried about competing with younger women for husbands. But today we feel the need to compete for men's attention in a work world where men still hold the majority of management positions.

Sadly, appearance discrimination is an embedded concrete reality: older and/or fatter women are systematically paid less and passed over for promotion. For example, researchers found that, among working adults in the US, "women are over 16 times more likely than men to perceive employment related discrimination and identify weight as the basis for their discriminatory experience."[13]

Knowing this, we may strive for a slender androgynous look, hoping to be taken seriously, rather than be judged by our bodies' sexual and reproductive qualities. Instead of mentoring and celebrating younger women who benefit from our pioneering in the workplace, we resent them—especially when they take weaker stances on women's issues or discount our contribution to their opportunity.

In addition, we haven't talked enough with each other and our male colleagues about successfully (and fairly) negotiating issues of sex, power, collegiality and communication on the job. Men often interpret a woman's energy, attention, or interactions as sexual. Simultaneously, we tend to hold women more accountable than men for sexual transgressions, making sexual energy in the workplace a challenge for women of all ages. These hotly charged attitudes and tensions infuse the workplace with self-doubt and confusion for many women.

Knowing how male colleagues may respond to our energy, we are understandably hesitant to initiate powerful, energized interactions—undercutting the authority we may need to succeed in business. Some male coworkers seek collegiality and friendship, but others manipulate sexual desire and energy to enhance their power.

These loaded topics are difficult to discuss openly in the workplace. Too often, we try to paper over complex office tensions by shaping our appearance and behavior to "please" the men we work with and for. That unhealthy diversion of our energies does nothing to confront the very challenges that men and women both face at work.

Retirement

Retirement looks a lot different than it did a generation ago. Some women's careers now last long enough to end with formal retirement. Other women keep working past "retirement age." Even if we improvise retirement as we go along, important life questions arise.

- What do we want to do now?
- How far can we go to explore the dreams, goals and interests that career diverted us from?
- Will that exploration disrupt other aspects of our life and relationships?
- Can we do something new or well without a boss or colleague's validation?
- What value do we have to our profession and community as a retired woman?

Retirement brings important logistical questions about the future. If we interrupted a career for childrearing and were (like many women) paid lower wages, do we have enough money to do retirement well? Do we sell the house? Start another career? We may feel inept and inadequate at managing money and IRAs, but skilled in the math of fat grams and calories.

Once again, however, intense attention on appearance obscures the more important (and more ephemeral) challenges like: "After decades of doing for others, do I have the right to wants or desires of my own?"

"Workplace Wellness"

Many corporate and government organizations have introduced wellness programs in recent years. Of course, it's great for employers to care about our well-being, but many of these programs focus on weight loss, dieting and exercise regardless of the individual's actual health status. Rewarded for engaging in weight loss and exercise contests to "promote health"—and penalized for not participating—employees with an eating disorder—or employees trying to recover—perceive employers encouraging and expecting symptomatic behaviors. Equating weight with health also puts people struggling with body image and self-regulation issues at risk.

Many of my patients have great difficulty practicing treatment and recovery skills—or focusing on their personal needs—while working where the corporate climate endorses diet talk and fitness frenzy.

Gail first came to me for treatment in her 40s after struggling with an eating disorder and depression her entire life. She used our time together well, working hard to believe that she deserved to take care better care of herself. But her low-paying, long-hours, no-benefits jobs limited how often she could come.

When she came back for treatment a decade later, she was exercising compulsively, counting calories, and eating poorly—a pattern triggered by her employer's wellness program. Drawn by the promise of a health insurance discount and pleasing her supervisor, she knew her behaviors were unhealthy. She won "wellness" awards at work but her dangerously low weight required a medical leave for intense treatment to get her back on track.

Another patient named Christy struggled with binge-eating. She reacted to her company's "Biggest Loser" contests by severely restricting her eating and exercising to the point of dizziness during the day, before returning home to binge intensely at night. Full of shame, Christy felt humiliated when she did not lose weight.

Without trained staff to guide the process and identify emerging medical problems, misguided "wellness" programs can create a toxic environment, promoting the problem of "perfecting" our bodies, as if it needed any extra help.

Women's Families

Child-rearing

Within moments of giving birth, a mother is responsible for feeding her child. Most of us hold feeding responsibility for the entire family—always within a few feet and a few hours of providing meals. That's quite a challenge if we feel conflicted about eating and food.

If we already struggle with body image issues, we may over-emphasize our children's appearance, clothes and shape as early as the toddler years. Sharing our adolescent daughters' interest in dieting, clothing, cosmetics, etc. may also be a form of intergenerational bonding—and add twists of intergenerational competition to an already knotty relationship.

We may also envy our children's emerging sexuality as we are suddenly surrounded by vibrant young people experimenting with and oozing sensuality. It's not unusual to feel subtle or overt urges to compete with our daughters, their friends, or our son's girlfriends, as we strive to demonstrate that we are still sexually attractive. Instead of "acting our age," we may dress like kids, sculpt our bodies, and over-exercise to prove our youthfulness and vitality. These behaviors foster annoyance and reciprocal competition from daughters—whose adolescence already supplies enough insecurity about appearance and social standing.

If our daughter develops an eating disorder, we may have intense trouble managing our own relationship to food and body. Many young eating disordered clients are followed into treatment by their mothers, who are unsure if they really deserve help. They struggle with guilt for having any needs of their own—even after suffering in silence for years.

Parenting itself provides stressors and disappointments for which we may not be prepared. Not every minute of mothering is exciting or rewarding, so we may feel like it doesn't "measure up" in our instant-gratification world. Our children's needs can be draining, monotonous, painful, and not at all like our romantic notions of what mothering would be like.

Resulting feelings of resentment, depression, or emptiness may lead us to use food to dull the pain. Or we may focus on our bodies as a means of control or accomplishment, just to feel that some part of our life is still ours alone. In contrast, when we honestly express our true hungers—and the complex emotions associated with being a mother—we aren't as apt to turn to eating problems or body image despair.

Single Parenting

Recently divorced and the 40-year-old mother of three, Martha was struggling with a whole array of eating disorder symptoms. She restricted most days, and then binged once or twice a week when her kids were with their dad and she felt empty and alone. She handled her guilt over bingeing by purging via exercise and laxatives. Every now and then, when she felt really desperate, she vomited.

When Martha came to me for treatment, she described how much she hated the vomiting, because it reminded her of high school, when her bulimia first began. That was a very dark time of her parents' severe marital conflicts and ultimate divorce, when Martha's symptoms felt totally out of control.

As Martha told her story, it was no surprise that she had relapsed into an eating disorder after her divorce. Martha explained that she'd promised herself she would never put her own kids through a divorce. So, she tried hard to have the perfect marriage, sacrificing much of herself to make her husband happy and to create a perfect home and family. When her husband had an affair, Martha blamed herself, convinced that her natural weight gain after three pregnancies was the reason for his infidelity.

Of course, the marriage's problems were more complicated than that. But Martha initially responded by dieting and losing weight to regain control of her life, and perhaps even rekindle her husband's romantic interest in her. Before long, she was in the midst of eating disorder chaos. However, she didn't see that right away. Restricting didn't seem like a problem (it felt like control); but the purging bothered her. She kept trying to convince herself that "it isn't so bad, because it isn't full blown bulimia." She justified the laxatives and the exercise as ways to cope with the bingeing.

Martha worked hard to keep her symptoms secret, bingeing and purging when alone. She did her best to continue to meet other people's expectations—and was good at keeping things perfect for everyone else, especially her children. In the meantime, she faced the stress of returning to a full-time career in the workplace after being the primary parent for a decade—and dating again after being in one relationship for nearly 20 years. Despite her belief she could control her symptoms, her life became a perfect mess before long.

One day, a close friend asked Martha how she was doing, gently suggesting that she seemed distant and disconnected. Martha trusted this friend enough to admit that she could no longer maintain the façade of perfection. The friend encouraged her to seek help and even came with Martha to the first therapy appointment.

In therapy, Martha and I focused on the deep disconnections she felt and how she could begin to deal with the pain of her divorce, the loneliness of being a single parent and the anger with her ex-husband. We talked a lot about her chronic perfectionism and how to begin to accept her needs and feelings, instead of seeing them as weaknesses or flaws. I also emphasized the need to take care of herself as well as the care she took of everyone else. Soon, Martha began to realize that her relapse reflected the impact of multiple life transitions she was experiencing as her marriage ended and life as a 40-something single mother began.

For instance, we discussed how reasonable it was for body image concerns to intensify as she reentered the workplace and the dating world. We explored how desperately Martha wanted to control something in her life during this time of major change, so she returned to familiar eating and appearance obsessions that she used to cope during her stressful adolescence. I suggested that her symptoms may also function to distract and redirect her anger about the divorce. She gradually became more able to accept and express anger that her perfectionism had never permitted.

Some single mothers, stressed by their multifaceted responsibilities, turn to managing their food intake and their weight in order to feel a sense of control. Ensuing compliments about weight loss and/or dedication to exercise may fleetingly fill an emotional void. Others will binge or eat compulsively using food to fill up and/or numb their emptiness. Unfortunately, these behaviors can prevent women from dealing directly with the complicated—and entirely normal—emotions associated with single parenting and ageing.

Like Martha, single moms often feel ashamed of "failing" in their relationships with their children's other parent(s). Added to the pressure to be the perfect single parent, attempts to perfect their bodies can be a coping strategy which locks these women in that lonely prison of perfectionism. With her friend's help, Martha escaped.

Deciding Not to Have Children

There have always been women who choose to forgo motherhood, like the generations of nuns who dedicate their lives to spiritual growth and serving the community. Some contemporary women avoid parenting out of fear of losing control of their weight, shape and "attractive" status after pregnancy and childbirth. Other women today make the childless choice for more altruistic and internal reasons. Regardless of our motivations, the decision is foreign and threatening to many people. As a result, adult women who choose not to be mothers endure exponentially more scrutiny and suspicion than adult men without children.

Friends and relatives may actually ask, "What's wrong with you that you don't want kids?" We may feel like round pegs being forced into square holes, struggling to feel okay about going against cultural expectations. Having such a deeply personal decision scrutinized by others can make any woman feel uncertain or uncomfortable. Even if we remain confident in our choice, we may not feel confident that others will accept and respect it as they should.

One way of fighting back may be "perfecting" our bodies to show that we are still young and free. Making our bodies impervious to criticism may seem an attractive solution to the complicated feelings of guilt and anxiety over how we may have disappointed others.

Empty Nest

Women derive much of our identity from parenting because the mother role is so deeply imbedded in our nature, our expectations for ourselves and the world's expectations for us. When our children leave home to launch their own adulthoods, our identity can feel threatened.

Life without daily responsibility for our children means developing a new relationship with ourselves and our future. It also means rethinking and readjusting our relationships with the kids, our partner and our community. We may ask the following.

- What is my role now that a central part of my womanly identity is over?
- What will happen to my marriage now that the kids aren't here to fill up all that space and use up all of our attention?
- Will I be interesting enough to my partner now?
- Will he or she be interesting enough to me?
- Do we stay in this home or move somewhere else?
- Is it time for to explore dreams, goals and interests that family responsibilities took me away from?
- Can I handle quitting my job or moving?
- What do I stand to lose if I do make major changes?

- Will life exploration or reexamination threaten my marriage or otherwise make me look at something I'm afraid of?

Because empty nest is such a major life change, it comes with a fair share of insecurity. Even if we couldn't wait to be released from being so needed by our kids, we may have forgotten how to have a relationship without being needed in that same intense way.

Directing time and energy toward making our outsides "look better" may appear easier than asking essential questions about our inner selves and our future. In addition, we can't help but think about aging, mortality and loss of attractiveness when watching our little babies morph into full-grown adults. Body obsessions may seem like the way to resist the passages of time and life.

Marriage of Children

Witnessing a child choose a life partner is a loss with a reward at its heart—an explicit example of joy and sorrow weaving together during life's important transitions. It is a beginning that marks an end, and an end that marks a beginning. Our family gets smaller as our child moves away from us, while simultaneously expanding with the addition of her spouse, children and in-laws.

Unfortunately, modern wedding preparations frequently focus instead on dieting schedules for mothers, bride and bridesmaids. This may trigger obsessions about looking young, fit and stylish at a stage in life when there is much to celebrate—including the natural beauty of aging, a child's life partnership and grandchildren. We may eagerly anticipate and intensely cherish our grandchildren, but never want to look like grandmothers.

Aging Parents

The demands of caring for aging or ailing parents are often considered an optional responsibility for men, but a requirement for women—with none of our other responsibilities taken away. As part of "the sandwich generation," we feel caught between fulfilling the needs of our children and our parents. It feels normal to believe that we're not sufficiently fulfilling our roles as spouse, child, parent, worker and community member— or securing enough time to recharge ourselves and grow. This addition without subtraction leaves us counting the ways we don't measure up or don't do things well enough, no matter how efficient we are.

Caring for an older parent can bring up unresolved issues from our childhood, reawakening the pain of old unmet needs. This can result in grief, anger and the disheartening feeling that we lack the bandwidth to address these lifelong conflicts in a productive way. On the other hand, the renewed daughter-parent contact provides the chance to work through the past, say, and listen to things that need to be said—ultimately making peace with our parents and our childhood.

Caring for our parents' aging bodies brings a vast array of powerful and painful emotions. Furthermore, we begin to confront the reality that our own bodies are aging and naturally losing capacities they once had. Eating and body image issues can easily emerge at these times.

Our desire to be forever young and healthy is easily stimulated while watching the demise of our parents' bodies. Vowing not to age as our parents did, or suffer the same illnesses, we may jump into obsessive and/ or pathological rituals of exercise and eating. These rituals appear to promise predictability during a difficult transition, but they also distract us from acknowledging the emotions stirred up as we care for, and then lose, a parent.

Women's Relationships

> If you think marriage is going to be perfect, you're probably still at your reception.[14]
>
> Martha Bolton

Infidelity and Desire

Sally was a "good girl" her entire life, always living dutifully for others— and especially to please her father. Even though she was now in her late 30s, Sally never permitting herself to acknowledge, let alone act on, any impulses aimed to please herself. Dieting and appearance were always important, but had never gotten out of control before. Sally looked like she had it all—a great education, exciting career, two children and marriage to a well-respected, equally accomplished guy named George. But her "perfect" persona was in fact disconnected from any real desire, happiness and self-satisfaction.

Sally was not prepared for the strong attraction she developed for Jeff, a colleague at work. In their high-powered, fast moving business environment, it was easy to get close to Jeff and allow a distance to grow with George. All of a sudden, Sally plunged deep into an extra-marital affair, feeling guilty and overwhelmed at her transgressions. She cared deeply about both men, but was ashamed and afraid of being discovered. So, she stopped eating to numb these feelings.

A close friend recognized Sally's weight loss and anxious mood, and convinced her to seek therapy. Gradually, Sally began coming to terms with the multiple reasons for her affair, deal more directly with these emotions, and make decisions about herself and her marriage. A pivotal moment occurred when I mentioned that the late 30s are usually the peak of a woman's sexual desire and satisfaction. This information normalized and legitimized Sally's feelings, helping her make sense of her affair.

Sally became much more aware of her own needs and feelings, allowing more room in her life and psyche for her true hungers. She and I labeled her weight loss as an ultimately positive event. It led her into therapy, which eventually gave her permission to appreciate her deepest appetites—and finally freed her to live without an external "script" for her future.

Women are often judged more harshly than men when it comes to infidelity or being "outside the box" sexually. A woman who is unfaithful is called (and may think of herself as) a slut, even if hers is a one-time infidelity.

This double standard reflects how little we respect, discuss, or even acknowledge the existence of women's sexual appetites. Even if we think grown men shouldn't act on adolescent "sow their wild oats" urges, we tend to resign ourselves to the fact that they will anyway.

From the earliest days of puberty, by contrast, we expect that girls should "just say no" to sexual desire. Boys who sleep around are studs, while girls who go to third base are whores. Girls seldom develop the power to say "yes" freely to their sexual appetites.[15] Many of us still don't know how to give a healthy "yes" as we reach our sexual peak in our 30s and 40s. Women young and old lack positive ways to express many desires and needs openly.

These same conflicted dynamics of desire occur in lesbian relationships, reinforced by cultural intolerance (despite legal recognition of same-sex marriage). Internalized homophobia can complicate our experience of trust and tension in intimate same sex bonds. Lesbians are not immune from falling back on the language of fat and body image distortion as a way to avoid dealing directly with relationship difficulties. My clinical experience indicates that lesbians who have to hide their true nature, identity and appetites are at greater risk of developing these problems.

We may embark on a sexual affair when we undergo a crisis about getting old or looking old. We may feel disappointed about not achieving perfection in our primary relationship —or even knowing how to ask for and get the intimacy we want. We may seek recognition from someone else:

• to prove that we are still attractive and desirable
• out of fear that our partner is losing interest in us
• because we feel smothered, not alive, and not appreciated in our family and marriage
• in reaction to lingering, unresolved issues with our parents
• to reclaim or find important parts of our self
• to have new or "perfect" sexual experiences.

It is very difficult to explore these issues while hiding an affair, or while being condemned if the affair is revealed. Becuase it requires a cycle of secrecy, infidelity can take us further away from addressing core questions about self, self-worth, purpose and desire.

Cultural double standards reinforce our shame while fostering disrespect for women's sexuality and discomfort with the notion that women have appetites of any kind. These distorted beliefs about our sexual desires provoke resentment against any urges and hungers—whether sexual, physical, or emotional—and encourage us to turn that anger against our body, the "source" of those unruly desires.

A Partner's Infidelity

When a woman's partner has an affair, it feels like an incredible body image failure: "He's out there because I'm not attractive or sexually enticing to him anymore." "She cheated on me because I'm inadequate." "It's all about my weight."

Many women believe that "perfecting" their bodies will win their partners back. This reaction can quickly kick into a pattern of exercise abuse, extreme dieting and other behaviors that threaten our health. Changing our appearance does nothing to address infidelity's violation of trust (the core of any intimate relationship) nor does it nurture the trust we need in any attempt to heal the relationship.

If our partner's crisis is related to getting or looking old, we may react by trying to appear young ourselves. If she or he is acting strangely or playing around, we may try to increase our feminine charms, resorting to a "sexy" façade rather than directly addressing how the crisis is affecting our him/her, us, and our relationship. In turn, we may react with stress, anxiety and depression—and then attempt to self-soothe through disordered eating or other body image obsessions.

Women are acculturated to take responsibility for other people's feelings. Therefore, we may overdo our help and discount our own needs, wants and desires when a partner goes through a difficult emotional stretch—like an affair or other midlife crisis.

Many women feel great ambivalence about whether we can we be angry about a partner's infidelity. We may stay stuck in sadness to cover over our anger. "If I want to make it better, how can I be mad? That might drive my partner away." As a friend once quipped, "depression is anger without enthusiasm." If we don't feel entitled to express our natural anger, it has to go somewhere; eating and body are visible and handy receptacles for it.

After an affair, we naturally (and reasonably) have a large load of distrust for our partner. But the crisis of trust triggered (or brought to the surface) by the affair *does* have the potential to ultimately strengthen our intimate bond. Repairing a post-affair relationship means a great deal of effort and usually professional help. It requires paying attention and dedicating courage, commitment and willingness to take risks. While "looking better" may be an attractive strategy, it isn't a solution.

Divorce

When we enter long-term relationships, we know that a staggering number of them end in divorce (our shorthand for the end of a long-term intimate partnership, whether or not it includes a state-sanctioned marriage).

Women are more likely to blame ourselves for this devastating loss, since we tend to take on more responsibility than men for the emotional work in an intimate relationship. So, on top of loneliness, sadness and anger over the end of this important relationship, we are likely to go through a period of serious self-criticism.

After divorce or separation, we feel inadequate and that we've profoundly failed at something women are supposed to know how to do instinctively: maintain an intimate partnership. Here are some common things divorcing women tell me in therapy.

- It was such a surprise. I always felt sure we would be together forever; everyone thought we were perfect together. What did I do to mess this up?
- I'm the first one in my family to get divorced. I've let down and disappointed my parents, my in-laws and all the rest of my family.
- Is there something wrong with me? Were the unmet needs in our marriage my fault? Was I expecting too much?
- I initiated the breakup; he didn't want it. I'm probably being way too selfish.

It's normal for divorcing individuals to feel traumatized and depressed by their situation. For many women, this means a case of the "Separation Skinnies." At first, the stress and shock may cause us to lose weight unintentionally. Soon we may start to feel good about this "accomplishment" (and the compliments we get) and begin more conscious efforts to lose more weight. Or, we may start overeating and bingeing in response to the strain and sadness.

Many of us put at least some blame for a divorce on our bodies. "If only I'd been more attractive, or stayed sexier, he or she would still be with me." But partners who seek sexy trophy brides are often acting out anxieties they can't seem to address directly. For example, they may fear getting old and dying.

We still teach young boys more about how to maintain what men's activist Jackson Katz calls a "tough guise" than we teach them about emotional literacy.[16] Boys often carry this handicap into adulthood and their intimate relationships. Shaping our bodies into something "too good for him to leave" does nothing to address that underlying problem. After all, no one can build a successful marriage on body parts.[17]

Divorce is difficult at any age, but it may be an especially profound loss to a woman who invested many years in a marriage, is older, feels less attractive, and does not want to be alone—or dating. The older we get in a youth- and appearance-focused world, the tougher it is to tolerate an "imperfect" physical shape that may not attract potential mates.

The rituals of excessive exercise, restricted eating, or bingeing can seem to supply structure to a chaotic time, although they don't provide the cohesion and schedule of an intimate human relationship. "I don't have to go home, so I go to gym" may seem like a good solution (and moderate exercise certainly helps with depression), but that approach quickly becomes hollow if body obsession is our primary approach to addressing the end of what we thought was a life-long relationship.

Post-divorce Parenting

After divorce, we often maintain a cycle common during marriage: taking responsibility for the relationships between our children and the other parent(s). Even if relations with an ex are fairly good, we often oversee his parenting, his difficulties and perhaps even his emotional life. We may remain the family "switchboard," managing the schedule and mediating between kids and Dad. This can be a matter of habit, guilt about the fallout from our breakup, and/or the conflicted and complex feelings we still have about our exes.

Successfully integrating stepparents (or their equivalents) into our children's lives is hard work. Of course, blended families can become bonus families,[18] but rushing into a new intimate relationship can make the journey harder.[19] Regardless of the timing, we'll need to learn new ways of communicating with our ex and leave responsibility for his/ her relationships in his/her hands. That includes relationships with our children and stepchildren.[20]

Meanwhile, we are living in a culture where "one" doesn't seem to be a whole number, so we may feel compelled to secure another mate immediately. Our culture over-romanticizes relationships and we can feel "wrong" or out of place if we're alone. Pressure to be part of a pair can also come from parents and family members. Plus, there is the natural desire for humans to partner with one another, a sense that may feel especially heightened after a previous relationship has ended.

Naturally, when we think about trying to find a partner, we start worrying about how we look. Our awareness of appearance and body image is heightened, not always in a good way.

But it is important to remember that one is a whole number. We can make valuable contributions to our families, friends and the world whether single or coupled.

> It isn't what happens to us that causes us to suffer; it's what we say to ourselves about what happens.[21]
>
> Pema Chödrön

The Common Thread

Any adult transition, change and challenge can bring loss, pain and uncertainty. It can also bring great excitement, vision, freedom and opportunity. Complicated by the pressure to be "perfect," developmental change can trigger body loathing, food obsessions, yo-yo dieting, life-threatening eating disorders, depression, addiction and more.

For women, the thread of body image weaves through every one of these issues. Most of the time, we either don't see the truth about weight and survival as we traverse the rough roads of adulthood, or else look at it through lenses that justify the pursuit of perfection rather than the pursuit of peace with an imperfect reality.

Loss Inventory

Think about one particular loss you experienced during adulthood: a death, health problem, change of status for you or your family, etc. The loss might obvious to others (death of a spouse) or more private and symbolic (your parents selling the house you grew up in).

As you remember that loss, jot down your answers to these questions.

- Have you talked about this loss with others?
- If not, what has stopped you from sharing it?
- If you have talked to others, how did you feel about their response?
- Have you received the support you need from others?
- Do you feel different as a person as a result of this loss?
- Has it changed your relationships? Brought you closer to anyone?
- Has it brought anything new into your life?
- How has it affected your sense of self and identity as a woman?
- How has it affected your attitude toward life?
- Has it changed your attitude toward your body?
- Do you pay more, less, or different attention to self-care and health as a result?
- When you initially experienced the loss, did you change your eating, exercise, or other body-related attitudes and behaviors?
- What is your body's typical reaction to stress and loss?
- Are there ways you could take better care for yourself during periods of loss and grief?
- How did you feel about answering these questions?

There are no right or wrong answers to these questions because we each respond to loss in our own way. There is no singular path toward healing and resolution. However, it is normal for the disruption of severe loss to upset the routine of our daily lives, including physical functioning and eating. We may eat more than usual, or temporarily lose our appetite. During these times of loss and transition, the best course is to maintain a physically healthy routine, especially when it comes to the basics of nutritional intake, sleep and exercise.

The Change Balance Sheet: What Are My Adult Transition Gains and Losses

Do this exercise by yourself, with a trusted friend, or in a small group. Write down your answers so you can reflect on them over time.

- What were the five most important things you gained during your 20s?
- What were the five hardest things to lose in that decade?
- Of these ten things, which two were the most important to your personal development, shaping who you are today? Do they come from the gain or the loss column?
- What was your emotional and spiritual state or condition during this phase of life?
- How important was your physical shape? Did it overshadow other things in your life? Did it overshadow your emotional and spiritual condition?

Repeat this exercise for each decade you've lived through:

- your 30s
- your 40s
- your 50s
- your 60s
- your 70s, and more if you are blessed with a long life.

What do your written answers reveal? What pattern or patterns do you recognize? Was one decade more challenging to your personal growth than another? What do your answers teach you about your adult development?

Notes

1   A 1917 poem in Edward St. Paige, *Zaftig: The Case for Curves* (Seattle, WA: Darling & Company, 1999) p. 122.
2   Anita Diament, *The Red Tent* (New York: Picador, 1998).
3   Carol Gilligan and Lyn Mikel Brown, *Meeting at the Crossroads: Women's Psychology and Girls' Development* (Cambridge, MA: Harvard University Press, 1992) and Gilligan, *In a Different Voice: Psychological Theory and Women's Development* (Cambridge, MA: Harvard University Press, 1993).
4   Helen Fisher, *The First Sex: The National Talents of Women and How They Are Changing the World* (New York: Random House, 1999) p. 185.
5   Germaine Greer, in Fisher, ibid., p. 182.
6   Quoted in Nancy Friday, *The Power of Beauty* (New York: HarperCollins, 1996) p. 494.
7   Ages on Inauguration Day, January 20, 2017. Fiorina born September 6, 1954 (https://en.wikipedia.org/wiki/Carly_Fiorina); Clinton born October 26, 1947 (https://en.wikipedia.org/wiki/Hillary_Clinton).
8   *The Change: Women, Ageing and the Menopause* (London: Hamish Hamilton, 1991) cited in Friday, op. cit., p. 507.
9   Ernest Becker, *The Denial of Death* (New York: Free Press, 1997).
10 In Gloria Wade-Gayles (Ed.) *My Soul Is a Witness: African-American Women's Spirituality* (Boston: Beacon Press, 1995) p. 181.
11 Kim Parker (2015). "Despite progress, women still bear heavier load than men in balancing work and family." Pew Research Center *Factank*. See www. pewresearch.org/fact-tank/2015/03/10/women-still-bear-heavier-load-than-men-balancing-work-family/ (retrieved August 14, 2015).
12 Personal communication with Joe Kelly, July 2003.
13 Mark V. Roehling, Patricia V. Roehling and Shaun Pichler (2007) "The relationship between body weight and perceived weight-related employment discrimination: The role of sex and race." *Journal of Vocational Behavior*, 71 (2), 300–318.
14 See http://www.marthabolton.com/html/speaking.html (retrieved January 28, 2016).
15 Joe Kelly, *Dads & Daughters®: How to Inspire, Support and Understand Your Daughter* (New York: Broadway, 2003) pp. 125–128.
16 *The Macho Paradox: Why Some Men Hurt Women and How All Men Can Help* (Naperville, IL: Sourcebooks, 2006).
17 Kelly, op. cit., p. 49.
18 See http://bonusfamilies.com/ (retrieved August 19, 2015).
19 See   http://bonusfamilies.com/bonus-living/new-relationships/   (retrieved August 19, 2015).
20 See www.joekelly.org/tips_for_live_with_moms (retrieved August 19, 2015) and Kelly, op. cit., p. 240.
21 See http://pemachodronfoundation.org/ (retrieved September 18, 2015).

3 Fact vs. Fiction

How Survival Shapes the Body

Show me a body part, I'll show you someone who's making money by telling women that theirs looks wrong and they need to fix it. Tone it, work it out, tan it, bleach it, tattoo it, lipo it, remove all the hair, lose every bit of jiggle.[1]

Jennifer Weiner

Every woman's physical shape has major implications for her survival. But these implications are quite different than you think.

Paradoxically, we live in an era of intense weight concerns *and* widespread myths about the importance of weight to our health. Even more problematic, most of us also hold misguided notions about a person's actual ability to alter and control her body's shape. So, before we go any farther, we have to learn the facts (and debunk the common fictions) about the connections between weight, health and body image.

For example, dieting seems like the logical, necessary response to eating too much or wanting to lose weight. However, science indicates that this conventional wisdom is completely backward: "To put it concretely, it is not bingeing that causes dieting, but dieting that causes bingeing."[2]

Such an assertion may seem absurd, but only because our cultural body myths ignore biological and genetic reality. Our personal experience bears that out—when we skip a meal or try to eat very little, we usually end up eating more later on. Hunger, left unsatisfied, doesn't go away, it grows.

We hear constantly that being "overweight" is risky to health and that everyone should lose weight. However, the truth is much more complex. Many women simply do not understand the connection between the shape of our bodies and the shape of our health.

Your body loves you. It's always operating to keep you alive. It makes sure you breathe while you sleep, stops cuts from bleeding, fixes broken bones, and finds ways to beat illnesses that might harm you. Your body loves you so much. It's time to start loving your body back.

Online meme[3]

In the next few pages, I'll knock down some of the most harmful myths by looking at scientific knowledge about the way the body works.

How Our Bodies Survive

The human body is hard-wired to respond quickly when confronted by starvation. The reason is simple: across the long history of the human race, starvation has been a serious threat to our survival, as it remains for millions of people around the world today. In order for the human species to survive, the body had to develop ways to survive as long as possible during food shortages.

No amount of technological or cultural progress changes how that works.

When calories and nutrition go missing, our bodies respond as if they are starving—because they are. Instinctively and almost immediately, the body responds to food deprivation by slowing down its metabolism, the rate at which it consumes calories (the units used to measure energy supplied by food).

The deceleration in our metabolism is a natural, primeval and unstoppable preservation response to *any* reduction in food intake; our bodies don't know whether a sudden change in its food supply is the result of famine, forgetfulness or a fad diet. It really doesn't matter; our bodies just want to keep us alive.

Nature also designed our sense of hunger to protect us from famine. When famine turns to feast, our bodies crave nutrition from the newly available food, and consume more than normal to make up for the recent deprivation. However, the body's metabolism ramps back up more slowly than hunger cravings do—because feasts are often sporadic and short-lived during times of overall famine. In this way, the body makes the new calorie supply last longer, just in case the feast fades.

The human body's speedy and innate ability to counter starvation is quite marvelous. The *female* body's survival capacity borders on miraculous.

Before puberty, a girl has about 12 percent body fat. During puberty, nature's hard-wiring multiplies her fat cells until she has sufficient body fat (about 17 percent)—to ovulate and menstruate safely. Natural female growth—uninterrupted by dieting—creates a mature adult body with about 22 percent body fat.[4]

That fat supply provides enough energy for an ovulating female to survive famine for nine months, the length of a full-term pregnancy. If faced with sudden food shortage or starvation, her metabolism will slow down, and she'll gradually consume the fuel naturally provided by fat cells. Through the hard-wiring of their bodies, pregnant women can survive a food shortage long enough to give birth—assuring survival of the human species for millennia. Nature also assures that women gain fat first in the breasts, buttocks, hips and thighs to protect our fertility, reproductive and feeding organs.

It may seem incredibly unfair that women need a higher percentage of body fat to be healthy than men do—and that men can lose fat more easily. But that's the way it is. And, as we can see, it is that way for a miraculously good reason.

The fat difference between men and women is not a weight issue or a character flaw; fat cell development is programmed into the female body by the internal wisdom of survival. Fat cells are our friends. In addition to ensuring survival, they produce estrogen to maintain bone density, decrease the risk for osteoporosis, and help us manage symptoms of menopause like sleep problems, hot flashes and complexion changes.

What's more: men are five times more likely to die during a famine than women.[5] That's good reason to be thankful for how women's bodies are designed to survive.

Dieting and Obesity

Obesity is a major public health issue today. However counterintuitive it may seem, a major root of obesity is dieting, not bingeing. Weight cycling (with its associated nutritional depletion, physical cravings and emotional deprivation) is a greater risk to our health than weight or body fat[6].

Researchers have known for decades that diets can't fool Mother Nature.[7] If we go on a diet, thanks to our evolutionary survival mechanisms, we will lose weight. For a while.

A few people sustain the weight loss, just like some lifetime smokers never develop cancer, but the odds are against it.[8] That's because our increased calorie intake is now entering a body still in precautionary metabolic "slow down" mode. No wonder nearly everyone who embarks on a food restriction diet eventually regains the weight she lost, and often gains additional weight.[9] Instead of saying a diet makes us lose pounds, it is more accurate to say the pounds go on vacation—bringing back new friends when they return.

Once we've regained the weight, most of us eventually try another diet. The same cycle repeats, with slightly greater extremes at each end. The more we yo-yo through diets over the years, the greater the extremes, and the more out-of-whack our metabolism and hunger cues become.

Meanwhile, the more diets we try, the more money we send to diet book publishers, pharmaceutical companies, herbal supplement manufacturers, "shaping" salons, gyms, spas, doctors and all the rest. The $60 billion-a-year US diet industry[10] has a big stake in keeping us on the yo-yo ride. Its false premises and false promises are perfectly good for profits, and perfectly awful for our psychological and physical well-being.

The "Skinny" on Food, Weight and Health

Contrary to a body myth that most people believe, no clear link exists between weight and health. Being perfectly thin doesn't bring well-being any more than having red hair does. For example, the mortality risks related to obesity have been grossly oversimplified.[11] The primary food-related mortality risk is poor nutrition, not a person's weight. Insufficient physical activity also increases mortality risk, but the health culprit is exercise habits, not weight.

Weight must be considered in context; separate it from other factors and we miss the picture entirely. For example, health problems among overweight US residents living in poverty may be due more to *being poor* than to *being fat*.[12] People in low-income neighborhoods have less access to healthy foods; more access to cheap, high fat foods; and may not be safe when engaging in outdoor physical activity, like walking or playing sports.

Myths about weight also distort perceptions about deeper traits, such as character, self-discipline and other moral qualities. Many of us continue to judge people (including ourselves) as "good" or "bad" by the standard of body shape, ignoring the immutable forces of genetic ancestry, internal metabolism and body chemistry.

By the way, heavier people don't always eat more; they may have slower metabolisms and a genetic code that gives them a higher body fat concentration. That genetic code may *also* leave them in excellent health, even if they weigh more than "average."

> I don't see how we're going to stop eating disorders [and other body image problems] until we stop reading character into the size of people's bodies. It's stereotyping. We've made progress against other stereotypes, and we can make progress against this one, too.[13]
>
> Deb Burgard

Unfortunately, weight prejudice makes it harder for heavy people to be healthy. For example, fat people often draw judgmental stares and comments on the street, at the gym, or in yoga class. The resulting discomfort and self-consciousness may suppress their activity level, and harm their health.

A widespread myth is that health is determined solely by the individual's behaviors. In fact, social, economic and environmental factors play a significant role. For example, poverty, stressful living environments and/or discrimination have real psychological health impacts.[14] Such chronic stressors cause changes in our hormonal and nervous systems, put us in a constant emergency state, and make us less likely to be able to engage in self-care and healthy behaviors. To assure a healthy country, we need to address both social and individual behavior influences.[15]

In addition to prejudging a person's integrity by her size, we also judge food itself through a thick and distorting veneer of morality. Depending on the latest sure-thing diet, carbs may be "good" this year while protein is "bad," regardless of the food's safety or quality. Next year it might be vise versa, but we'll still rigidly adhere to the misguided moral classification of food. The things we eat become weighted with meaning, power and value beyond what they deserve.

So, let's set aside the myths and live with the facts. Weight and health are not the same thing. Food is food. If you're allergic to peanuts, then peanuts are risky ... not evil. Our arteries will suffer if we eat nothing but cake, but that doesn't make it "bad." In fact, frosted cake could be perfect for your next birthday.

Spare Tire or Life Preserver?

As her metabolic rate declines 15 to 20 percent, the average menopausal woman will gain 12 to 15 pounds, usually settling around the waist (just like it does for men around the same age).[16] While those fuller fat cells make pants and skirts fit differently, they also generate natural estrogen to reduce the severity of our menopause symptoms and post-menopausal problems like bone loss. Our lower metabolism rate helps keep this valuable fat in place.

Unfortunately, obesity concerns have many health care providers promoting midlife weight loss, without regard for the potential implications. If we diet our way through pre-menopause, perimenopause, and menopause, we stop reinforcing our diminishing stores of natural estrogen, and risk more dramatic and distressing menopausal symptoms.

When we diet during midlife, our remaining fat cells must strain harder to make up the estrogen deficit left by "lost" fat cells. Paradoxically, this makes the remaining fat cells stronger, more stubborn, and much harder to eliminate through dieting—one more example of how nature protects our bodies.

So, despite our pursuit of perfect abs, a bit of "spare tire" is *good for us* as we move into menopause.

Concerned about an underlying eating disorder, a well-attuned primary care physician referred a woman in her early 70s to me. Barbara did not think she had an eating disorder, but was open to talking about the role eating plays in managing stress. She began to see a clear connection there, recognizing how she lost weight at key transitional times in her life. I shared information about how our fat cells begin to get larger and produce estrogen during menopause to help us avoid osteoporosis and other problems. At the next session, she walked in with her arm around her waistline, announcing: "I used to think this was a spare tire. Now I know it's my life preserver!"

Barbara learned to accept that her body had innate knowledge about how to protect and care for her. Appreciating her thicker middle, she began exploring her emotional life and needs through therapy. Eventually, Barbara no longer needed to restrict her eating to feel in control of her life and she regained the weight that she lost. Her health improved and she restored her usual level of vitality and excitement about life.

Here's the ultimate problem: underweight women *die* earlier. A nine-year study of 5,200 women and men over 65 found that higher body mass index (BMI) is associated with lower mortality rates in older adults.[17] Another eight-year study of 8,029 predominantly white women aged 65 and older found similar results. These researchers concluded:

> Our results do not support applying the National Institutes of Health categorization of BMI from 25 to 29.9 kg/m² as overweight in older women, because women with BMIs in this range had the lowest mortality.[18]

A review of multiple studies indicates that extra weight may actually bring women other benefits by reducing the risk for illnesses such as lung cancer, premenopausal breast cancer and osteoporosis.[19] For example, thin women had the greatest risk for lung cancer, while obese women were much less likely to develop it. This doesn't mean that we should necessarily try to gain weight; however, if our weight is low because we are restrictive in our eating or excessive in our exercise, we may put our overall health at risk. Weight and health are extremely complex issues; one does not necessarily bring the other.

The Shape of Genetics

It is fairly common for women to read and hear—or to tell ourselves— that we should lose five or ten pounds after the holidays. Few, if any, of us ever read, hear, or tell ourselves that we should grow five or ten inches taller after the holidays, or any time of year. The notion is absurd because we know that we can't change our height.

Just like our height, and the color of our skin, eyes and hair, our general body shape and size are genetically shaped. To a great extent, our genes determine our weight, distribution of body fat, skeletal frame, basic metabolism and appetite. If your ancestors were short and skinny, your chances of being short and skinny are great. The same principle applies if your ancestors were tall, fat, dark skinned, pale skinned, diabetic, alcoholic, or prone to sickle cell anemia.

Let's assume that you don't have a chronic illness, endocrine problems, or genetic abnormalities. If you eat a balanced diet and engage in aerobic activity (not easy in a world of junk food, 500 TV channels and continuous online streaming), you'll fall into the healthy weight range determined by your heritage and genetic code. Dieting throws that natural balance out of whack, which is why nearly every dieter eventually regains all her "vacationing" weight along with additional pounds.

Note that we did *not* say that you will reach your ideal or perfect weight. Each of us has a genetically pre-determined, perfectly natural weight *range* that our mature bodies seek to maintain.[20] Because nature defaults to a balanced mode, many adults maintain a stable weight without really paying much attention to it, while most dieters find themselves back at their original weight.

The myth that we have (and should rigidly maintain) a perfect weight ignores the human body's essential flexibility and its natural developmental process. For instance, we are hard-wired to burn more calories on days when we eat more, and to burn fewer calories on days when we eat less. Scientific research has repeatedly proven this phenomenon. There is no "perfect weight," no fixed number of pounds that is "right" or genetically immutable.

The term Body Mass Index, or BMI, is used frequently in discussions of weight and obesity, but actually has no relevance to an individual's health. Based on the relation between one's weight and height, BMI was developed to track population trends. As with the weight tables which insurance companies developed decades ago, science shows little connection between BMI and health.

For example, in 1998, the National Heart, Lung, and Blood Institute changed the BMI at which we are deemed "overweight" from 26 to 25, instantly moving millions of Americans from the normal weight to the overweight classification, even though nothing about their health had actually changed.[21]

The revised agency guidelines for "normal weight" (a BMI of 18.5–24.9) contradict other government studies. For example:

- a BMI of 25 is associated with the lowest death rate for white men and women
- a BMI of 27 is associated with the lowest death rate for African-American men and women
- Native-Americans with a BMI between 35 and 40 do not have an increased risk of death despite being more than 10 points above "normal"
- a BMI of *less than* 20 is associated with a higher mortality rate.

These confusing and contradictory uses of BMI numbers lead many women into weight reduction regimens that are far more dangerous than the pounds they carry.

Alternative (and more rational) BMI guidelines have been proposed by eating disorders experts like Marcia Herrin. Her framework reflects the underestimated risks of low weight and the exaggerated risks of higher weight, while accounting for the many gender-based physiological differences between men and women. Herrin's guidelines for women are shown in this table.

Health Status	BMI range (kg/m²)
Risky low weight	Below 18.5
Low weight	18.5–19.9
Minimum safe weight	20–24.9
Safe weight	20–29.9
Risky high weight	Above 30

Herrin defines minimum safe weight as "the lowest weight at which a person can maintain healthy functioning (including regular periods for women and normal testosterone levels for men), meet nutritional needs, and not engage in eating disordered behaviors and thinking."[22]

The bottom line: as women age, there is no established relationship between moderate weight increases and increased health risk. So we need to pay less attention to calculating our body's relationship to gravity, and more attention to nurturing healthy human relationships, giving ourselves adequate food, exercising wisely and finding emotional balance.

> Let the world know you as you are, not as you think you should be, because sooner or later, if you are posing, you will forget the pose, and then where are you?[23]
>
> Fanny Brice

Surviving Womanhood

Many women with eating disorders say that they were showered with compliments about their shape and their self-control at the same moments that they felt physical and emotional chaos, afraid that they were about to pass out or even die. These "compliments" confuse, dismay and interfere with getting help—sometimes until it is too late.

Audrey was a successful writer and activist working with a nonprofit promoting girls' well-being. She battled bulimia and anorexia for more than ten years, but received short-term treatment on only a few occasions, because insurance did not reimburse for more than a few treatment days, and there were no inpatient treatment programs in her state.

Audrey's symptoms were intensifying again when, as part of her job, she flew across the country to attend a conference on eating disorders. On the plane, Audrey felt strong heart palpitations, and feared that she might have a heart attack and die, but she said nothing to her colleagues, some of whom were in recovery from eating disorders.

By the time she returned home, Audrey was frightened because her symptoms weren't abating. Desperate for help, she finally decided to enter the nearest eating disorders treatment program, several hours drive away. While waiting for admission, she continued working and trying to survive how horrible she felt. One evening, she went out with friends, who lavished praise on Audrey for how thin she was and how good she looked.

Back home that night, Audrey asked her fiancé, "How could they think I look good? I feel miserable, desperate and like I could die. I'm completely confused." She was right to wonder about her friends' perspective, and to fear the intensity of her symptoms. Less than a week later, on the day before she was to enter treatment, Audrey had a heart attack and died.

Audrey's friends are not to blame for her illness or death. They were not hard-hearted or mean-spirited. Like most of us, culturally induced perfectionism distorted their perspective about the importance of female appearance, leaving them blind to their friend's reality. Our culture embeds this warped value system deeply into our individual ways of seeing the people and situations around us. We believe that a woman who looks good must feel good and *be* good, because she has the moral fiber to obtain the perfect female beauty ideal: thinness. We believe these things even if they bear no relation to the particular woman's suffering.

The perfectionistic mindset amplifies cultural attitudes to reinforce body image paradoxes and conflicts. Women have new authority in the world, but we still feel undermined by our beautifully imperfect bodies.

- When was the last time we were part of an all-woman conversation where *no one* brought up weight, food, or personal appearance?
- Even with career success, why do we still scan other women in a room, to see how we stack up in the "obligatory" weight and appearance competition?
- Liberation from old gender stereotypes brings new independence and choices, so why do we spend more time on fad diets than figuring out how to share work-family balance struggles?
- Why do we talk more about our body imperfections than we do about our spiritual well-being?

In the last few pages, we've debunked some deeply entrenched body myths. But the facts about genetic and biological realties have a hard time sinking into our collective consciousness. We live in a culture that continually and convincingly sells the fiction that we *can* perfect our bodies.

But even temporary alterations of the body cannot change immutable realities like a parent's death or a child's march toward adulthood. As Jennifer, Audre, and Naomi's stories illustrate, our external shape can mask the actual state of our psychological, spiritual, emotional and physical lives—disrupting our most important human relationships. If perfecting our bodies is our first (or only) response to life's transitions, then we are living a myth that distorts our lives today and in the future.

Exercise: What Happens When We Diet to Lose Weight[24]

How We Diet	*Results of Diet*
Skip meals or decrease calories	• Metabolism lowers, making fat easier to store from fewer calories. • The body's need for fuel causes rebound "munchies," usually for high fats and sugars. • Hunger causes poor attention span, irritability, fatigue, muscle loss.
Cut out starches	• The body loses a source of stable energy, increasing moodiness and fatigue. • The body's need for fuel causes rebound "munchies," usually for high fats and sugars.
Cut out meats	• Risk of iron deficiency leading to fatigue. • Energy from meals does not last as long, so cravings increase for between-meal high fat, high sugar foods.
Preplanned meal replacement diet or liquid diet	• Muscle mass loss accompanies fat loss. • Metabolism slows, making it easier to store fat on liquid calories. • "Quick-fix" plans don't develop lasting healthy eating habits.
Fasting	• Water loss accounts for most weight loss. • Muscle mass decreases. • Lowered metabolism results in fat gain. • Prolonged fasting is associated with many health problems, including fatigue, headache, dehydration, dizziness, constipation, hypoglycemia, anemia, muscle weakness and gallstones.
To be slim	• In 95 percent of cases, "lost" weight is regained within two years; this prompts more restriction cycles, with similar results. • Yo-yo dieting can lead to obesity.
To be healthier	• Dieting cycles increases health risks. • Being plump has health benefits (especially for midlife women), while there is evidence that being too slim is unhealthy. • Dieting can decrease muscle mass necessary for good health.

How We Diet	Results of Diet
	• The body and mind don't run well on restricted calories/energy.
	• Mood swings, irritability, and food obsession increase as *physiological* responses to starvation.
To be more attractive	• Genuine friends and loved ones value who we are, not how we look.
	• Successful long-term relationships can't be built on body shape.
	• Dieting is a self-centered activity.
	• Mood swings, irritability, and food obsession are unpleasant to be around.

How many of the results in this table did you know about already? Did any of the results surprise you?

Notes

1 "Great! Another Thing to Hate About Ourselves." *New York Times*, February 12, 2015, SR4. See www.nytimes.com/2015/02/15/opinion/sunday/from-sports-illustrated-the-latest-body-part-for-women-to-fix.html (retrieved September 18, 2015).

2 Janet Polivy and Peter C. Herman (1985). "Dieting and binge eating: A causal analysis." *American Psychologist*, 40 (2), 193–201.

3 This meme was popularized online in 2014 and 2015 by Richard Williams, better known as the rapper Prince Ea. While frequently attributed to Mr. Williams, neither his office nor the authors have been able to find an original citation.

4 Debra Waterhouse, *Like Mother, Like Daughter: How Women are Influenced by Their Mother's relationship with Food and How to Break the Cycle* (New York: Hyperion, 1997).

5 Debra Waterhouse, *Outsmarting the Female Fat Cell After Pregnancy* (New York: Hyperion, 2003).

6 Kelley Strohacker and Brian K. McFarlin (2010) "Influence of obesity, physical inactivity, and weight cycling on chronic inflammation." *Frontiers in Bioscience*, E2, 98–104.

7 Kathy Kater, *Real Kids Come in All Sizes* (New York: Broadway, 2004) pp. 138–139.

8 Linda Bacon and Lucy Aphramor, *Body Respect: What Conventional Health Books Get Wrong, Leave Out, and Just Plain Fail to Understand about Weight* (Dallas, TX: Ben Bella Books, 2014).

9 Traci Mann, Janet A. Tomiyama, Erika Westling, Ann-Marie Lew, Barbara Samuels and Jason Chatman (2007) "Medicare's search for effective obesity treatments: Diets are not the answer." *American Psychologist*, 62, pp. 220–233.

10 See www.worldometers.info/weight-loss/ (retrieved August 14, 2015).

11 See Berg, *Women Afraid to Eat* and Gaesser, *Big Fat Lies*.
12 Bacon and Aphramor, op. cit.
13 Mary Duenwald, "Body and Image; One size definitely does not fit all." *The New York Times*, June 2, 2003. See www.nytimes.com/2003/06/22/health/body-and-image-one-size-definitely-does-not-fit-all.html (retrieved August 12, 2015).
14 Thomas E. Fuller-Rowell, Gary W. Evans and Anthony D. Ong (2012) "Poverty and health: The mediating role of perceived discrimination." *Psychological Science*, 23 (7), 734–739.
15 Bacon and Aphramor, op. cit.
16 "Weight gain during menopause." See www.34-menopause-symptoms.com/weight-gain.htm (retrieved August 12, 2015).
17 Ian Janssen, Peter T. Katzmarzyk and Robert Ross (2005) "Body Mass Index is inversely related to mortality in older people after adjustment for waist circumference." *Journal of the American Geriatrics Society*, 53 (12), 2112–2118. See www.medscape.com/viewarticle/518415.
18 Chantal Matkin Dolan, Helena Kraemer, Warren Browner, Kristine Ensrud and Jennifer L. Kelsey (2007) "Associations between body composition, anthropometry, and mortality in women aged 65 years and older." *American Journal of Public Health*, 97 (5), 918.
19 Sandy Szwarc (2007) "News women can use." See http://junkfoodscience.blogspot.com/2007/04/news-women-can-use.html (retrieved August 12, 2015).
20 Bacon and Aphramor, op. cit.
21 Sally Squires, "Optimal weight threshold lowered." *The Washington Post*, June 4, 1998, A1. See www.washingtonpost.com/wp-srv/style/guideposts/fitness/optimal.htm (retrieved August 12, 2015).
22 "The new improved BMI." *Psychology Today*, posted March 26, 2015. See www.psychologytoday.com/blog/eating-disorders-news/201503/the-new-improved-bmi (retrieved October 10, 2015).
23 In Norman Katkov, *The Fabulous Fanny* (New York: Alfred A. Knopf, 1953) p. 101.
24 Adapted from Margo Maine, *Body Wars: Making Peace with Women's Bodies* (Carlsbad, CA: Gürze Books, 2000).

4   The Shape of Eating Disorders

But I am learning that perfection isn't what matters. In fact, it's the
very thing that can destroy you if you let it.[1]

Emily Giffin

In the months following Anna Westin's death from anorexia, her parents
became outspoken advocates for access to eating disorders treatment and
for education to prevent them. One evening Anna's mother, Kitty Westin,
attended the premier screening and reception for a PBS documentary
about eating disorders treatment. After the screening, one of the anorexic
patients profiled in the film took questions from the audience alongside
her physician. The crowd was overwhelmingly female, and nearly all the
questions asked the woman for very specific details about her dieting
patterns and obsessive exercise. Kitty recalls:

> It was bizarre and disturbing. You figure these women have some
> awareness and concern about the plague of eating disorders;
> otherwise they wouldn't be at a screening for this film. But here they
> were asking things like, "How far did you run every day? I know
> that got to be a problem for you, but how far do you think it would
> have been OK for you to run? By the way, you know, I think you look
> great!"
>
> Most of the questions amounted to asking "How far can I go with
> your techniques so I can be sure to lose weight, but not slip over
> the edge into anorexia?" They were belittling the disease that was
> consuming this brave woman onstage and that killed my daughter.
> Even after seeing a documentary on the horrors of eating disorders,
> they seemed blind to how obsession with weight was already eating
> up their own lives, and blind to how their eagerness to uncover the
> "techniques" of bulimia and anorexia might endanger them—and the
> young woman onstage.
>
> How could this be when the damage was staring right at them in
> the person of this young woman trying to answer their sick questions?
> She was clearly struggling with her own pain and the horrific stories in

the film—while simultaneously hurt and confused by how eagerly the audience sought to learn the "tricks" of her pathology. I was furious.[2]

Seduced by the Shape

I tell Kitty's story for a very pointed reason. The intense personal and cultural pressure to attain a perfect body creates deeply mixed feelings about eating disorders and their symptoms. Even if we don't engage in these behaviors, we may feel drawn to use them to "perfect" our own bodies. We may think the following.

- I can figure out a way to work just a few anorexic tactics into my life, because it clearly helped anorexics lose weight; those women just went too far.
- I'd only do a few of those things, and only to get myself to a better weight.
- It really would make me feel good, and I wouldn't go far enough to get into trouble.
- The only thing keeping me from the perfect body is effort, the right formula and willpower.
- I'd only vomit up meals occasionally, especially when I eat "forbidden" food.
- That time I went a few days without eating, I lost more weight than ever, and people kept complimenting me on how good I looked.
- One of my colleagues at work is probably bulimic. Maybe I can ask her how she does it, and then copy her just a little bit. It seems to work for her and I'm sure I can control it.

Those seductive thoughts are dangerous, even if they seem normal to us. Acting on these thoughts is not normal, healthy, or safe—no matter how often our culture seems to endorse them, and no matter how many women around us seem to share them. Even the thoughts themselves, without any action, are dangerous. They sap our energy, distract us from more important things in life, affect our mental health, and can make it easier to slip subconsciously into patterns of behavior that endanger our physical health.

Women with eating disorders and body image obsessions never anticipate how much suffering will eventually result from starting down their destructive path. They don't set out to cause themselves and their loved ones pain. They start down this road because they are trying to deal with difficult and inconvenient emotions, and meet life's challenges by pursuing a perfect body—they don't go down it looking for a dead end. But a dead end is, figuratively—and sometimes literally, what they find.

Disordered eating may "work" in the short run, giving us a sense of power and control or helping us feel more attractive to others, but it doesn't solve the underlying problems. Our body is not the journey or the destination. It cannot ultimately determine the shape of our life and happiness.

When people learn that I specialize in eating disorders, they often tell me, "I'd like to have anorexia for just a week or two, so I could lose some weight," or "I just want to be bulimic when I eat too much and feel stuffed." Sometimes I'll reply:

> Well, cancer and chemotherapy also make people lose weight. Even if it were possible, would you like to have cancer for just a week or two? Eating disorders and body image obsessions are no different from other serious illnesses. It isn't wise to joke about them or pretend that they can disappear on command or be easily cured. Nor should we wish them on ourselves or others.

Even when they don't end a woman's life, eating disorders steal years of it. What follows is the only demand I will make of you while reading this book: as we go through the rest of this chapter, I want you to reject the belief that you (or anyone else, including me) are above or immune from eating disorders. We can't dabble in pathological behavior and expect to keep it under control. If or when we play with *this* fire, we *will* get burned. If this chapter upsets, frightens or distresses you, consider seeking help, even if you don't think you have a textbook eating disorder.

What are Eating Disorders?

> And so, to be fat is to deal with people's projections that you are a loser, whether you feel like one or not; and, to be thin is to live in fear of exposure of your inner loser-ness. Clearly, changing one's body size provides no solution to the existential question of how to claim one's imperfection as a human being.[3]
>
> Deb Burgard

Eating disorders are detectable illnesses that affect the sufferer's physical, psychological, spiritual, emotional and relationship life. They are not a passing fad or the fashionable *illness de jour* of the rich and famous. Modern medicine has recognized eating disorders for many years as diagnosable, life-threatening conditions suffered by people (overwhelmingly women) of all socioeconomic classes. This isn't a new phenomenon either; in centuries-old documents, medical historians find regular mention of symptoms that are recognized today as eating disorders.[4]

Calling this type of illness "eating" disorders can easily misdirect us from some important truths. Eating disorders *involve* food and eating (or not eating), but they are not really *about* eating. It may help us think more clearly about eating disorders if we just call it the Perfect Problem. The central issue for a woman with eating disorders is how she feels about her life, the pressures she feels to prove her self-worth, and the destructive behaviors and attitudes she employs to try to feel some sense of self-worth. An eating disorder is the perfectly distorted answer to the self-doubt contemporary culture creates for women.

For women in our culture, proving our worth is tangled together with the fear of being fat, or not thin enough. Self-image entangles with cultural attitudes to foster fat phobia, weightism and "thin-itis," thereby normalizing and validating unhealthy and hazardous practices. Because our culture fosters these dangerous behaviors, we have difficulty knowing the difference between what is healthy and what is pathological.

The shape and progression of eating disorders change as women age. Some women recover from severe eating disorders in their youth but still have subclinical obsessions with their eating or appearance (which means having some, but not all, of the symptoms that indicate a full-blown eating disorder).

A study of 45- to 64-year-old Canadian "weight preoccupied" women indicated a higher incidence of bingeing, feeling guilty after eating, feeling out of control of food, and giving too much time and thought to food than younger women report.[5] Meanwhile, the percentage of adult women seeking inpatient eating disorders treatment rose from 4.7 percent in 1989 to 11.6 percent in 2006.[6] Unfortunately, weight preoccupation, perfectionism and eating disorders don't disappear with age.

Older women's symptoms may change over time, morphing into exercise abuse, over-control of their or their family's food intake, constant anxiety and rumination about their body and appearance, obsessive shopping, or repeated cosmetic surgeries. Because these habits seem normal in our culture, they are harder to recognize than, say, severe anorexia. Therefore the problems go unidentified by us, our health care providers, or our loved ones. Meanwhile many adult sufferers wonder if they need or deserve help because they no longer fit the clinical teenage stereotype of someone who has an eating disorder.

Like alcoholism, an eating disorder is not caused by a failure of morality or willpower. It is a real, treatable medical illness in which certain maladaptive patterns take on a life of their own. These serious disturbances in eating behavior include extreme reduction of food intake, severe overeating, purging and over-exercise and distress about body shape or weight. Researchers have yet to nail down exactly how and why initially voluntary behaviors, like dieting, develop into an eating disorder for some people, but not for others.

Types of Eating Disorders

Although we describe specific eating disorder diagnoses below, some clinicians and researchers use a "transdiagnostic" approach, appreciating the common ground across and among identified eating disorders—instead of focusing on the differences.[7] In the transdiagnostic paradigm, all eating disorders emanate from the same faulty beliefs about self-worth and the importance of controlling weight, shape and appearance.[8] Many patients present with different sets of symptoms at different points—sometimes more anorexic, other times more bulimic, and still others with a mixture of symptoms (see OSFED later in the chapter) or with binge-eating.[9] My adult patients have often moved from one symptom cluster to another over the course of their lives so recognizing the disorders' transdiagnostic, or shared, features makes sense to me.

Anorexia Nervosa

People with anorexia nervosa can look in a mirror and perceive themselves as fat even when they are dangerously thin.[10] Eating becomes an obsession involving abnormal habits, like weighing food and keeping a strict account of caloric intake. A woman with anorexia may skip meals entirely; eat only certain foods (and those only in small portions); weigh her body obsessively; exercise compulsively; vomit; and use stimulants, laxatives, enemas and diuretics in misguided attempts to lose weight.

A woman struggling with anorexia often denies that she has a problem, and may develop elaborate excuses, rationalizations and behaviors to convince herself and others that nothing is wrong. Her self-worth and sense of self are determined primarily, if not exclusively, by her body shape. She has an intense fear of becoming fat and will resist eating normally or maintaining an average weight for her age and height. Her ovulation and menstruation may be disrupted or may cease altogether.

Some people fully recover after a single episode of anorexia. Some go through fluctuating patterns of weight gain and relapse. Others slide steadily down a chronically deteriorating course of illness over many years. Among all mental illnesses, anorexia has the highest mortality rate. The most common causes of death are cardiac arrest, electrolyte imbalance and suicide.

The longer a woman suffers from an eating disorder, the more likely she will have severe medical problems—or die. For example, five percent of women with anorexia are likely to die after enduring five years of the illness; after twenty years with anorexia, the mortality rate increases to between 15 and 20 percent.[11] Alcohol abuse among women with eating disorders increases mortality risk and is associated with deaths related to both medical deterioration and to suicide.[12]

While the threshold for serious medical problems and death is different for each person, our bodies can only take so much abuse. Since our bodies are less resilient as they age, adult women play a dangerous game engaging in eating disorders or other unhealthy behaviors.

Faced with the chronic food restriction of anorexia, the body eventually starts consuming the fat and then breaks down the muscle in vital organs like the heart, causing irreversible damage and, sometimes, organ failure. The disease also consumes self-worth and breaks down the vital psychological will to live, which is why many women with eating disorders commit suicide.

Here are some common health risks associated with anorexia nervosa:

- abnormally low blood pressure, which means that the heart muscle is weakening; the risk for heart failure rises as heart rate and blood pressure levels sink
- muscle loss and weakness
- severe dehydration
- kidney failure
- reduction of bone density (osteoporosis), which results in dry, brittle bones that are more likely to fracture, causing other health problems
- irregular and/or absent menstrual periods
- infertility
- fainting, fatigue and overall weakness
- dry hair, dry skin and hair loss
- growth of a downy layer of hair called lanugo all over the body, including the face, in an effort to keep the body warm (lanugo is the hair a newborn has for warmth but quickly loses)
- increased anxiety, depression and irritability
- poor concentration and obsessive thoughts about food, weight and appearance
- increased self-doubt and sensitivity to rejection
- premature death.

Anorexia nervosa is a frightening and stubborn illness. Researchers are still examining the numerous contributing factors and searching for more effective ways to treat and prevent it. There is no quick-fix for anorexia, but most sufferers will recover with proper care.[13] However, recovery takes an average of five to seven years—sometimes much longer—and is rarely a straight path.

Bulimia Nervosa

A woman with bulimia engages in a cycle euphemistically called bingeing and purging. As with anorexia, bulimia's symptoms include being in strong denial, often having a distorted perception of body image, and the sufferer deeply believing that her body shape and weight determine her worth.

A woman with bulimia will compulsively and repeatedly eat excessive amounts of food over a short time. She feels out of control during these binges. After a binge, she will take extreme steps to keep from gaining any additional weight from consuming all that food.

These steps include self-induced vomiting; obsessive exercise; extreme fasting; and abuse of laxatives, enemas, diuretics and other drugs. Bulimic bingeing and purging are almost always done in secret, and sufferers usually go to great lengths to hide their behavior. They are ashamed and disgusted with themselves while bingeing and purging—even though the behaviors may bring temporary emotional release, relief, and/or a numbing of feelings.

A woman with bulimia may be harder to recognize than one with anorexia. Since people with bulimia continue to eat, they often fall within or above the normal weight range for their age and height. However, they share the anorexic's fear of gaining pounds, obsessive desire to lose weight, and deep dissatisfaction with their bodies.

The health consequences of bulimia are very serious and include:

- electrolyte imbalances that can lead to irregular heartbeats, cardiac or respiratory arrest and premature death; this is due to the loss of potassium and other nutrients from the body as a result of purging behaviors
- inflammation, tearing and possible rupture of the esophagus from frequent vomiting
- tooth decay and staining from stomach acids released during frequent vomiting
- chronic irregular bowel movements and constipation as a result of laxative abuse
- muscle aches, fatigue, dizziness and a general sense of malaise
- increased self-consciousness, self-doubt, depression, isolation and shame
- loss of concentration
- increased emotional volatility
- irregular or absent menstrual periods.

Clinicians officially diagnose bulimia when the patient is bingeing and purging at least once a week for three-months or longer. A significant number of women alternate between bulimic and anorexic periods during the course of their illness.

Some women attempting to recover from anorexia have difficulty controlling or accepting new, healthy eating patterns, so they resort to purging, especially if they are not receiving adequate professional help. Similarly, some women with bulimia use anorexic behavior to cut their caloric intake severely as they try to avoid purging. There is more commonality than difference between bulimia and anorexia, especially in how they keep sufferers from dealing with shared fundamental issues.

Clinical experience shows that many underlying issues are common across ethnic lines, as well as between sufferers of one type of eating disorder and another. However, the ways particular eating disorders are expressed may vary. For example, African-American women may be more likely to purge with laxatives than with vomiting; West Indian women may use Epsom salts or other purgatives; Native American or Latino women may be more likely to overeat and then severely restrict, and so on.

Binge Eating Disorder (BED)

People with BED have frequent episodes of driven, out-of-control eating, similar to the bingeing seen with bulimia. The difference is that people with BED do not usually purge after a binge. Because they don't purge excess calories, many people with BED gain weight over the years. The disease and cultural prejudice against fat people combine to produce intense feelings of self-disgust and shame in BED sufferers. This often leads to renewed cycles of binge eating.

A woman with BED eats large quantities even when she doesn't feel hungry, eats more rapidly than normal, and/or eats until she is painfully full or falls asleep. An official diagnosis of BED requires bingeing once a week for three months or longer.

The health risks of BED are closely associated with the risks of clinical obesity. They include:

- high blood pressure
- high cholesterol levels
- heart disease
- diabetes
- gallbladder disease
- depression.

More men have BED than any other eating disorder, which makes sense, considering common male and female attitudes and fears. When it comes to body image, men are more afraid of being small and women are more afraid of being big. Hence the male drive to bulk up and the female drive to diet.

Other Specified Feeding or Eating Disorder (OSFED)

Previously known as "eating disorder not otherwise specified" (EDNOS), OSFED describes serious and real eating disorders that are related, but not necessarily identical, to anorexia, BED, or bulimia. According to the American Psychiatric Association, OSFED includes atypical anorexia nervosa, low frequency bulimia nervosa, low frequency binge-eating disorder, purging disorder in the absence of bingeing, and night eating syndrome.

The OSFED diagnosis is necessary because many women display some signs of anorexia, or bulimia, or both, but they do not meet all the diagnostic criteria for either one. Still, these women are suffering severe physical and psychological problems and face serious health risks. For example, they may have lost a significant number of pounds but still be in the normal weight range.

Others may purge without bingeing, or they may purge less often than the frequency required to diagnose bulimia. Others may chew food and spit it out; they don't vomit, but they don't swallow what they eat either. Although discussed less frequently, OSFEDs wreak just as much havoc in the lives of the women who suffer from them and bring many of the same physical and psychological dangers as other eating disorders. Some will actually have poorer outcomes and higher mortality rates than patients with anorexia or bulimia.[14]

Compulsive Eating

While binge eaters consume a large amount of food quickly, in a very driven manner, compulsive eaters may instead graze throughout the day, eating unconsciously and without regard to hunger. These behaviors evolve into the compulsive eater having a negative body image and feeling shame and embarrassment, which further isolates the individual from social supports, and makes food more important than ever.

Compulsive eaters can be any shape and size. This eating pattern usually causes weight gain, but some sufferers also abuse exercise or diet often enough that their weight stays within the normal range, or yo-yos up and down in a predictable range. Still, the sufferer's distress regarding their bodies overwhelms their self-image, and erodes their quality of life.

> Compulsive eating is basically a refusal to be fully alive. No matter what we weigh, those of us who are compulsive eaters have anorexia of the soul. We refuse to take in what sustains us. We live lives of deprivation. And when we can't stand it any longer, we binge. The way we are able to accomplish all of this is by the simple act of bolting—of leaving ourselves—hundreds of times a day.[15]
>
> Geneen Roth

Although not a formal diagnosis in the psychiatric manual, compulsive eating can pose the same physical threats as BED, as well as intense negative emotions in feeling that one's eating habits are out of control. A compulsive eater feels deep distress about her eating, self-image and self-esteem, and may try to compensate with numerous diets or fasts.

Too often, women with BED or compulsive eating are simply seen as having weight problems, and are referred to diet programs, which seldom work. Recovery and alternative coping mechanisms depend upon understanding the underlying emotional issues of self-worth and identity that build up and manifest themselves in food obsessions.

Orthorexia

Clinicians see an increasing number of patients who compulsively use and abuse health food or compulsively consume so-called alternative foods. Although also not yet recognized as a medical diagnosis, this behavior is known as orthorexia, which means "fixation on righteous eating." If a woman with orthorexia doesn't have access to her specific foods, she becomes extremely anxious and feels out of control. For her, health food takes on a much greater meaning.[16]

Steven Bratman, M.D., credited with coining the term orthorexia, acknowledges that most people could benefit from being more attentive to the quality of the food we eat. However, people who develop orthorexia have the opposite problem: they take the concept of healthy eating to obsessive lengths and paradoxically endanger their health.

We are bombarded with contradictory media reports about the healthy and unhealthy qualities of certain foods. Indeed, highly processed foods do contribute to a number of health problems. All this information sometimes feels overwhelming as we try to feed ourselves and our families. But concern about food can mushroom into something greater, especially as we get older and worry more about our health, youth and beauty.

Orthorexics are health food junkies who actually become emaciated as fewer and fewer foods seem acceptable to them—or when they can't easily obtain health food, especially when traveling away from home. The so-called raw food movement often fosters orthorexia and its practitioners can become deficient in protein, fat and other essential nutrients. Some orthorexia patients have orange-tinted skin when they start treatment; by eating too many fruits and vegetables, they get "too much of a good thing" like carotene.

Initially a lifestyle choice, an obsession about health food can become as serious as anorexia or bulimia. Orthorexia interferes with the quality of life, contributes to depressed moods and anxiety, causes social isolation, and even shortens life expectancy. Despite the similarities between orthorexia and other eating disorders, the motivation for orthorexia is different.

The strongest desire for most people with anorexia, bulimia and related disorders is to lose weight and change their appearance. In orthorexia, the first desire is to be pure, healthy and natural. (The desire for purity can also affect people with other eating disorders.) As we'll see in Chapter 8, recovery depends on understanding the multiple motivations underlying eating disorders.

Subclinical Eating Disorders

Psychologists and physicians have devised specific guidelines for diagnosing anorexia, bulimia, BED and OSFED. However, physicians and psychologists recognize that eating disorders occur along a continuum. Some women develop symptoms with less frequency and/or severity than a clinical eating disorder; but the symptoms still harm their quality of life.

Of course, purging and severe food restriction are not natural or healthy, even if they don't rise to the clinical definition of bulimia or anorexia. Even though the behaviors are subclinical, they still cause anxiety, sadness and negative feelings. They also cause physical problems, including gastrointestinal disruption, an impaired immune system, osteoporosis and generally poor health. As of yet, we do not have scientifically reliable estimates of how many people have subclinical eating disorders, but most professionals in the field are concerned that the problem is growing, and see many cases that eventually develop into full-blown eating disorders.

A 2014 study examined the prevalence of eating disorders in Austrian women aged 40–60. Researchers found that 4.6 percent met the full criteria for a clinical eating disorder and another 4.8 percent met the subthreshold standards. However, *both* groups reported the same degree of psychopathology, distress and impairment.[17] This suggests that even subclinical eating disorders have a significant impact on the well-being of adult women, and require professional attention.

Symptoms of subclinical eating disorders are similar to those for diagnosed eating disorders, but they occur with less frequency or intensity. A sufferer may switch between symptoms, and go through stretches of eating normally. With that distinction in mind, the signs of subclinical eating disorders include:

- counting calories, fat grams, or carbohydrates every time she eats
- chronic restrictive dieting
- exercising obsessively in order to burn up calories consumed
- skipping meals as often as possible
- trying to go days without eating
- repeated weigh-ins
- using laxatives, diuretics, diet pills, or other other-the-counter medications to lose weight
- wishing she was anorexic or bulimic
- engaging in some anorexic or bulimic behaviors, although inconsistently
- feeling guilty if she allows herself to enjoy food
- alternating between periods of excessive control and excessive indulgence with food
- cooking for others but not eating
- maintaining many rules about good versus bad food

- feelings of sinning, being immoral, or being bad when eating a forbidden food
- smoking cigarettes, chewing gum, or drinking coffee, soda, or water to avoid eating
- obsessively anticipating what food will not be eaten or how calories eaten will be burned up.

We could argue that these behaviors are normal for Western women. Unfortunately, we'd be correct, which is a frightening reflection on our culture (see Chapter 7). The biggest health concerns arise from repetition of these behaviors, and the level of emotional investment we make in them. When women with subclinical eating disorders feel overwhelmed by adult stressors, some will slip down into the pit of fully diagnosable eating disorders.

So is dieting *always* an early warning sign of a potential eating disorder? One quick test is whether we stop dieting once we reach our goal. Diets are unpleasant because success depends on constantly depriving ourselves. Therefore, on many levels, the desired conclusion of a diet is to end it as soon as possible and not subject ourselves to another one. But if we never stop these dieting cycles, or if we equate dieting with self-control and moral strength, our diets may warn of something more serious. Our food deprivation may be masking other issues.

Remember that undereating actually lowers metabolism, so dieting usually ends up adding weight. The average woman today diets more often and more rigidly than she did 30 years ago but weighs more! Between the slower metabolism and the rebound eating that follows most diets, it is very easy to gain weight, continuing the cycle of body image despair, poor nutrition and shame.

A Self-Assessment Tool

The table below is a simple way to get a preliminary idea of where you are in your relationship with food and eating. Fill in this table alone, at a time when you won't be interrupted. Read each statement, and fill in the response that best reflects how you feel and think right now. Be honest with your responses; no one will judge you on your answers.

Before tallying your responses, acknowledge how you felt while taking this assessment and how you feel afterward.

	Never	Monthly	Weekly	Daily	Multiple Times a Day
I read about dieting or weight loss obsessively.					
I make excuses for not eating.					
I skip meals intentionally.					
I try to go as long as possible without eating.					
I diet or restrict my food intake.					
I avoid social situations that involve food.					
I eat secretly.					
I have strict rules about food.					
I believe that some foods are good and some are bad.					
I only feel safe eating certain foods.					
I obsess about food.					
I feel guilty or ashamed if I break my rules about food or eat something I didn't plan.					
I worry about my weight.					
I watch what others eat and compare my intake with theirs.					
I chew gum or suck on hard candy to avoid eating.					
I smoke cigarettes to curb my appetite, avoid eating and maintain my weight.					
I drink diet soda, coffee, tea, or water to avoid eating and feel full.					
I cook for others but refuse to eat those foods.					
I count calories, fat grams, protein grams, or carbohydrates.					
I use food to reward or punish myself.					
I feel out of control of my eating.					
I exercise only to lose weight.					
I take laxatives, diet pills, diuretics, metabolism boosters, or other supplements to control my weight.					
I have had irregular menstrual periods or infertility problems.					

Look at the pattern of your responses. If most responses are in the Never or Monthly category, your eating concerns are probably manageable and do not interfere with the quality of your life. The more you checked Weekly, Daily, or Multiple Times a Day, the greater the probability that you have an eating problem. Talk this over with a trusted friend and consider making an appointment with a therapist who specializes in diagnosing and treating eating disorders. Your feelings alone may indicate whether you are suffering unduly and would benefit from some form of therapy.

Beyond Eating Disorders: Body Image Distress

> Because she is forced to concentrate on the minutiae of her bodily parts, a woman is never free of self-consciousness, She is never quite satisfied, and never secure, for desperate, unending absorption in the drive for a perfect appearance ... is the ultimate restriction on freedom of mind.[18]
>
> Susan Brownmiller

Despair, dissatisfaction and shame about the body are not the exclusive domain of women with diagnosable eating disorders. Many readers who do not yet see themselves described in this chapter may still battle body hatred on a regular (if not constant) basis. In fact, some problems related to body image are so severe that they reach the level of diagnosable disorders themselves.

This may be hard for most women to believe. After all, many of the symptoms we will discuss seem like a routine part of our everyday lives. However, they only seem typical because the pursuit of perfection and our culture's impossible standards for women *normalize* body image despair. Sadly, this normalcy doesn't diminish the harm. In fact, body image struggles can infect our lives and become so incapacitating that they require intense psychological intervention.

Body Dysmorphic Disorder

This psychiatric term describes preoccupation with an imagined defect in our appearance or an exaggerated reaction to a slight "imperfection." Someone with body dysmorphic disorder (BDD) overreacts or reacts uncontrollably (that is, pathologically) to moles, freckles, acne, minor scars or skin discoloration; hair on her face, body, or head; and the shape and size of breasts, muscles, or genitalia.[19] One or more of these supposed defects can trigger significant emotional distress and erode our overall ability to function normally. People with BDD avoid social situations and often develop other problems like depression, anxiety and phobias.[20]

Ironically, even the rare women who meet today's narrow definition of beauty often don't feel beautiful or adequate, because body image is not a rational thing. For example, some actresses and models admit to having BDD, because their body images are also constructed on the insecurity and self-doubt endemic to a culture that constantly assaults women with unattainable images of beauty and achievement.

BDD includes the following behaviors:

- repetitive mirror gazing or avoidance of mirrors
- obsessive grooming
- obsessively using clothes or make-up to conceal real or imagined flaws
- repeated medical visits to dermatologists or plastic surgeons to treat the perceived problem
- constantly comparing your appearance to others' appearance
- constantly fishing for compliments or reassurance about appearance.

These symptoms look like pretty normal behaviors for most women in a culture where entire industries like cosmetics, fashion, magazines, beauty, fitness and even areas of medicine are built on the premise that something is wrong with us that we must change immediately.

So if these behaviors are normal, how can they constitute a disorder? Doesn't "disorder" suggest *ab*normal? In a sense, it does. But medicine and psychiatry refer to a disorder as being a sickness, disturbance, or disease. The level of discord seen in body dysmorphic disorder is unnatural; it disturbs the norms of nature. Unfortunately, the same discord is often the norm for women in our culture. The logical conclusion is this: our cultural norms are themselves disturbed and disordered.

> Step away from the mean girls … and say bye-bye to feeling bad about your looks. Are you ready to stop colluding with a culture that makes so many of us feel physically inadequate? Say goodbye to your inner critic, and take this pledge to be kinder to yourself and others.[21]
>
> Oprah Winfrey

Chapter 7 will explore this cultural contradiction in more depth, but meanwhile let's take a simple example. Many cultural norms apply more often to women than they do to men, and vice versa. Therefore a simple way to examine the underpinnings of a cultural norm is to imagine applying it to the opposite gender.

Let's try it. Imagine a *man* who engages in:

- repetitive mirror gazing or avoidance of mirrors
- obsessive grooming
- obsessively using clothes or make-up to conceal real or imagined flaws
- repeated medical visits to dermatologists or plastic surgeons to treat the perceived problem.

Sadly, some men do have body dysmorphic disorder. Researchers studying men and women with BDD found:

> The men were significantly older and more likely to be single and living alone. Men were more likely to obsess about their genitals, body build, and thinning hair/balding; excessively lift weights; and have a substance use disorder. In contrast, women were more likely to obsess about their skin, stomach, weight, breasts/chest, buttocks, thighs, legs, hips, toes, and excessive body/facial hair, and they were excessively concerned with more body areas. ... Women also had earlier onset of subclinical BDD symptoms and more severe BDD as assessed by the Body Dysmorphic Disorder Examination.[22]

It may strike you as odd that some men have BDD. On the other hand, we usually *expect* the same behaviors from women. Our body obsessions seem normal and pass without comment. For example, many of us don't even let our lovers see us unprotected by a 24/7 armor of make-up and coiffed hair. Many of us will only be intimate in the dark, because we are afraid or ashamed of being seen naked even by our own closest partners.

Perhaps this is why some women feel relief at being diagnosed with BDD; it helps make sense of their obsessions, releasing them from feeling isolated and freakish. Self-consciousness, self-scrutiny and self-doubt are part of the body image norm that envelops nearly all women in Western culture.

Exercise Abuse

Exercise can be an effective and enjoyable stress reliever and a source of solace, achievement and strength. It can also become a way that women punish themselves for feelings of inadequacy. Many of us exercise primarily to change our bodies, not to enjoy them.

Adult female celebrities like Oprah Winfrey, Demi Moore and Cher have dedicated a large portion of their waking hours to rigid exercise regimens that are overseen by personal trainers. Younger generations of stars also live as though success and riches require exercise frenzy in pursuit of the perfect body. If we believe magazines and talk shows, these are the women we should emulate, making fitness one more area where we fall short of the female ideal.

Exercise abuse is exactly what it sounds like: mistreatment of our bodies through physical exertion. Too much exercise combined with too little nutritional intake can push the body into a dangerous slowing of metabolism that lowers all of our body's basic functions, like pulse, blood pressure and temperature. This state, called hypometabolism, disrupts the body's enzymatic reactions and immune system, making us more vulnerable to bacterial, fungal and viral infections. It produces symptoms like anxiety, depression, intolerance for heat and cold, hives, dry skin, hair loss, unhealthy nails, insomnia, fluid retention, asthma, fatigue, headaches, irritability—and reduction in ambition, motivation, sex drive, concentration and memory. A slowed metabolism also makes it harder to lose those hated pounds, so we have to exercise more to reach our goal, continuing the downward spiral.

> Perfectionism is self-abuse of the highest order.[23]
>
> Anne Wilson Schaef

Exercise abuse also leads to overtraining syndrome, which brings physical exhaustion, diminished performance, fatigue, stiffness, aches and pains and a general lack of strength. It can also result in chronic injuries such as torn muscles, ligaments, or tendons, stress fractures and even osteoarthritis. If we are not eating well, recovery from these injuries takes much longer. As fat stores become depleted, muscle tissues are also laid waste. In extreme cases, or when we put additional stress on the body (for example, from using laxatives, diet pills, or purging), exercise abuse can bring on cardiac problems and sudden death.

Here is a list I created to help my patients tell the difference between healthy exercise and excess exercise.[24]

- I judge a day as good or bad based on how much I exercised.
- I base my self-worth on how much I exercise.
- I never take a break from exercise, no matter how I feel or how inconvenient it is.
- I exercise even though I am injured.
- I arrange work and social obligations around exercise.
- I cancel family or social engagements to exercise.
- I become angry, anxious, or agitated when something interferes with my exercise.
- I know others are worried about how much I exercise, but I don't listen to them.
- I always have to do more (laps, miles, weights) and rarely feel satisfied with what I have done.
- I count how many calories I burn while exercising.
- I exercise to compensate for eating too much.

While exercise can be a very positive way to diffuse difficult feelings or manage stress, our hours at the gym or track can become addictive distractions, preventing us from addressing our emotional, relational and spiritual shape. If exercise is our only coping mechanism, we open the door to abusive excess exercise, sliding from self-discipline into self-destruction. Our bottom line question about fitness should be: Is my fitness goal to *be* strong and healthy or to *look* good?

A Warning to Athletes: Not Eating Can't Help You Win

Poor nutrition and low caloric intake undermine the purpose of exercise, even for athletes. It wastes training time, depresses metabolic rate, and can lead to serious eating disorders.

When food and fluid intake are too low, athletes experience the following.

Poor training benefit
- Energy intake is too low to meet training demands.
- Carbohydrate intake is too low for optimal recovery from training.
- Fluid intake is too low to rehydrate optimally after training.
- Performance shows minimal or no improvement.

Early fatigue
- Low muscle glycogen levels limit the body's capacity for high-intensity exercise.
- Dehydration limits exercise and impairs body temperature regulation.
- Low iron stores increase risk of anemia and compromise work capacity.

Reduced muscle strength, muscle endurance, speed and coordination
- Weight loss reduces muscle mass.
- Muscle is broken down to provide fuel for movement.
- The body is less able to meet training demands.

Low blood sugar
- Less ability to concentrate.
- Poor judgment and decision-making ability.
- Feelings of hunger, fatigue, light-headedness.
- May precipitate overeating, followed by guilt and sometimes by purging.

Increased risk of injury and illness
- Stress fractures.
- Respiratory illness.

Extended recovery time after injury or illness

Feelings of inadequacy, anxiety, anger, irritability, depression and loneliness

Perfect Pills

Women spend billions each year on pills, supplements and other products in hopes they will magically eliminate weight and reshape our bodies. Some widely used supplements turn out to be quite dangerous, even though they are benignly packaged and sold as health products at drug stores, nutrition centers, health food stores and internet sites. Others are totally ineffectual and harmless, except to our pocketbooks and psyches, since we want so badly to lose weight. These drugs are seductively marketed to seem like the answer when nothing else seems to help.

Most over-the-counter diet drugs and appetite suppressants contain caffeine and/or amphetamines (central nervous system stimulants). Both substances can generate jitters, anxiety, headaches and sleeplessness—not to mention their addictive potential. Depending on the drug's potency and the body's reactions, our hearts can race too fast, causing cardiac problems, heart attacks and even death.[25]

That's why diet drugs are for use *only* in extreme cases and when *closely monitored* by a physician.[26] However, many of us take these heavy drugs lightly—and repeatedly.

Women often use products designed for another purpose (like laxatives) in an attempt to shed pounds. Over-the-counter cathartic laxatives like Dulcolax® can be very dangerous when used in excess, depending on the ingredients and how our bodies react to taking them.[27] In addition, cathartic laxatives actually produce little real weight loss, because our bodies absorb most nutrients and calories at higher levels of the gastrointestinal system. Instead, laxative abuse can (and does) cause dehydration followed by rebound water retention.

Abusive cycles of laxative-induced dehydration and rebound water retention cause distressing weight shifts that keep the cycles going. Bloating leads to feeling fat; this leads to more laxative use, which leads to dehydration and then more rebound water-retention bloating, and so on. This dangerous cycle creates chemical changes that can lead to electrolyte imbalances, cardiac arrhythmias, heart attacks and even death.

Some women respond to body image distress with near-religious pursuit of extreme measures like colonics and fasting. At colonics retreat spas we easily pay $3,000 a week to not eat and empty out our systems.[28] Popular (and profitable) diet products and services change each season, with something new always being offered as *the* magic weight-loss formula. But we stubbornly refuse to learn our lesson, while the purveyors feed their wallets by feeding our culturally crippled body image.

Meanwhile, be forewarned: the US Food and Drug Association does *not* review or approve over the counter dietary supplements before they go on the market. Only after a pattern of problems is reported will FDA regulators study a product and *may* act to remove it, but this can come after deaths have already occurred.[29]

When it comes to diet products, remember the old folk definition of insanity: doing the same thing over and over again, but expecting different results. The pursuit of perfection is risky.[30]

Cosmetic Plastic Surgery

Attitudes about plastic surgery have changed dramatically. Fifty years ago, the stereotypical plastic surgery patient was a vain, self-centered and wealthy older woman with too much time and money on her hands.

Nowadays, elective cosmetic surgery is considered almost as normal as visiting a hair salon. The American Society of Plastic Surgeons reports 15.1 million cosmetic procedures in 2013.[31] Women accounted for 91 percent of those procedures; the most frequent ones being breast augmentation, nose reshaping, eyelid surgery, liposuction and facelift. Almost three-quarters of the people obtaining these operations were over 40:

- 17.2 percent were performed between on people aged 30 and 39
- 49 percent were performed on people between age 40 and 54
- 25 percent were performed on people aged 55 and over.

Let's be clear: what we're discussing here is *aesthetic*, cosmetic surgery, not reconstructive plastic surgery that repairs *medical* problems like cleft palate or a radical mastectomy. The American Society of Plastic Surgeons defines "elective surgery" as "action to proactively manage signs of aging or [to] enhance appearance." If that sounds like marketing language, it is. Plastic surgeons make their biggest profits when people choose to have surgery; we spent over $12.6 billion this way in 2013.[32] Without so-called aesthetic surgeries, the pool of patients remains limited to people needing medically necessary reconstructive procedures.

The pursuit of perfection creates an imperative that we redesign our natural shape, despite our records of actual and meaningful achievements.

When we buy into this cultural requirement, the costs are immense.

- We live by the bigoted and false rules that our body's natural shape and appearance should determine how important we are and how seriously we should be taken.
- Attempts to "perfect" our body's natural shape and appearance drain our mental, emotional and spiritual resources.
- Even without the psychological price, the balance sheet racks up billions of dollars spent on beauty products and procedures that don't (and usually can't) live up to their promises.
- While we spend (for example, over $55 billion annually on cosmetics[33]), companies plow our money back into advertising to

convince us that skin cream and hair dye can soothe our souls and solve the "problem" of aging.

• We risk losing our grip on who we are. Some of my clients are so afraid to be seen without these layers of protection that no one knows what they truly look like.

Of course, the widespread currency of these notions does not stop it from being absurd—and untrue. Our psychological and emotional well-being is not dependent on removing part of our stomach, chemically peeling our skin, or implanting synthetic sacs in our breasts.

It used to be that women were considered narcissistic, unstable, or—at the very least—neurotic if they wore heavy make-up all the time or took radical steps like plastic surgery to change their real appearance. In today's climate, these same women are viewed as motivated and achievement oriented. Modern plastic surgery campaigns promote breast enhancement as safe, effective and essential to women's mental health—just as they promoted breast *removal* as good for women's well-being in the 1920s, when the boyish flapper look was in style.

> If women suddenly stopped feeling ugly, the fastest growing medical specialty [elective cosmetic surgery] would be the fastest dying.[34]
>
> Naomi Wolf

Meanwhile, the pressure to be perfect contributes to cultural homogenization of beauty and to growing insecurity among non-Caucasian women about their body image. The positive trend of cultural diversity in media and advertising paradoxically complicates and intensifies issues about body image. For example, there is far greater diversity of body size and skin color among well-known male African American actors and models than there is among female ones (contrast Samuel L. Jackson and Halle Berry). Especially in advertising, the black women most likely to appear are the ones with the lightest skin and the most "white" facial and body features.

This "white" aesthetic infects the self-image of non-celebrities as well. By 2013, just over a quarter of cosmetic surgery patients in the United States were people of color.[35] This trend depletes the essential cultural asset of real diversity. The homogenization of beauty—and the belief that a manufactured body is better than a real one—undermines respect for the countless ethnicities, religions and races that enrich, and are essential to, the very life of our culture.

Women who engage in plastic surgery also pass a deficit on to their families. Children of cosmetic perfectionists may not have a sense of how their own bodies should naturally look as they age—or even recognize earlier pictures of their parents in the family photo album.

Despite the multitude of downsides, patients tell me that they see body-altering procedures as comparable to coloring their hair—an ordinary experience for an ordinary woman on an ordinary day.

Plastic beauty is not beauty at all, but it's the logical outcome of a culture that degrades and ignores older women and their wisdom.

> My limbs work, so I'm not going to complain about the way my body is shaped.[36]
>
> Drew Barrymore

During her first therapy session, an intelligent, attractive adult woman named Elaine told me that she finally got motivated to stop vomiting after deciding to have her "eyes done." Elaine explained that she did not want to waste the money she'd spent on the surgery, and she knew that if she continued to vomit, the results wouldn't last. Unfortunately, instead of vomiting, Elaine started restricting her food intake and abusing laxatives. Despite being an interesting, educated and accomplished woman, Elaine never sought help for these problems until it was almost too late; she nearly died after over thirty years of self-inflicted body abuse. Clearly, neither surgery nor disordered eating behaviors helped Elaine confront and resolve her core problems.

Does cosmetic plastic surgery ever help women struggling with issues about body image? Not if they have eating or body dysmorphic disorders. In one study, 83 percent of women with Body Dysmorphic Disorder had either no improvement or an increase in their distress after electing to have cosmetic surgery.[37] In another more recent study, the number was 93 percent.[38] Women with eating disorders often have *increased* body image disturbance after cosmetic plastic surgery, because the core issues that resulted in the condition are still present.

Now that we've described the havoc and damage that can result from eating and body image disorders, it's time we asked who is at risk, why those women start down this dangerous road, and why it is so difficult for them to change direction.

The Shape of Your Body Image

Is body image distorting the shape of your life? Look at the chart opposite and do this exercise alone, at a time when you won't be interrupted. Read each statement, and fill in the response that best reflects how you feel and think right now. Be honest with your responses; no one will judge you on your answers.

Before tallying your responses, acknowledge how you felt while taking this quiz and how you feel afterward.

	Never	Monthly	Weekly	Daily	Multiple Times a Day
I am ashamed of how I look.					
I compare my looks to other people's.					
I dissect my body into its parts instead of feeling at one with my whole body.					
I associate thinness or physical perfection with happiness, success and self-control.					
I call myself fat, ugly, or gross aloud or in my thoughts.					
I am certain that others see me as fat or unattractive.					
I believe that life will be better if I lose weight, fit into a smaller size, or correct my body's defects.					
I dismiss, disregard, or disparage compliments from others.					
I feel unable to enjoy life because of my body shape or appearance.					
I feel dependent on what others say about my appearance but still feel unable to believe anything positive they say.					
I am preoccupied with my weight.					
I hate my body.					
I dress in styles to hide my body.					
I am never satisfied with my appearance.					
I avoid social situations because of how I feel about my body.					
I will not wear a bathing suit or other revealing clothes in warm weather.					
I hate certain parts of my body.					
I consider having cosmetic plastic surgery.					
I want to be thinner than my friends.					
I hate the mirror.					
I repeatedly check myself in the mirror.					
I exercise only to lose weight.					
I get irritated if others say I exercise too much.					
I cancel social plans to exercise.					
I panic if unable to exercise.					
I base my self-esteem and mood on my appearance.					

Look at the pattern of your responses. If most of your answers are in the Never or Monthly category, your concerns about body image are probably manageable and do not interfere with the quality of your life. If most of your answers are in the Weekly, Daily, or Multiple Times a Day categories, that may be a warning sign that body image constitutes more than its share of your self-image. Talk this over with a trusted friend and consider making an appointment with a therapist who specializes in eating disorders and/ or body image distress. Your feelings alone may indicate whether you are suffering unduly and would benefit from some form of therapy.

Take inventory of how deeply these thoughts and beliefs intrude into your psyche. Consider ways to rework those thoughts and beliefs so you can free up energy for you and the things that will truly bring you happiness (more on this in Chapter 10).

Notes

1   *Something Borrowed* (New York: St. Martin's Press, 2004) p. 317.
2   Personal communication with Joe Kelly, 2003.
3   Debora Burgard (2010) "What's weight got to do with it? Weight neutrality in the health at every size paradigm and its implications for clinical practice." In Margo Maine, Beth Hartman McGilley and Douglas Bunnell (Eds.), *Treatment of Eating Disorders: Bridging the Research–Practice Gap* (London: Elsevier, 2010) p. 23.
4   Richard Gordon, *Eating Disorders: Anatomy of a Social Epidemic—Second Edition* (Hoboken, NJ: Wiley-Blackwell, 2000).
5   Jungwee Park and Marie P. Beaudet (2007) "Eating attitudes and their correlates among Canadian women concerned about their weight." *European Eating Disorders Review*, 15, 311–320.
6   Diann M. Ackard, Sara Richter, Maria J. Frisch, Deborah Mangham and Catherine L. Cronemeyer (2013) "Eating disorder treatment in women forty and older: increases in prevalence over time and comparisons to younger patients." *Journal of Psychosomatic Research*, 84, 175–178.
7   Christopher G. Fairburn, Zafra Cooper and Roz Shafran (2003) "Cognitive Behaviour Therapy for eating disorders: A transdiagnostic theory and treatment." *Behaviour Research and Therapy*, 41, 509–528.
8   Stanisław Malicki, Paweł Ostaszewski and Joanna Dudek (2014) "Transdiagnostic models of eating disorders and therapeutic methods: The example of Fairburn's cognitive behavior therapy and acceptance and commitment therapy." *Annals of Psychology (Roczniki Psychologiczne)*, 17 (1), 25–39. See https://tnkul.pl/files/userfiles/files/RPsych2014nr1pp025-039_Dudek_Ostaszewski_MalickiEN.pdf (retrieved August 20, 2015).
9   Gabriella Milos, Anja Spindler, Ulrich Schnyder and Christopher G. Fairburn (2005) "Instability of eating disorder diagnoses: Prospective study." *British Journal of Psychiatry*, 187, pp. 573–578.
10 Unless otherwise noted, material for descriptions of specific eating disorders is drawn from decades of clinical experience; American Psychiatric Association, *The Diagnostic and Statistical Manual of Mental Disorders, Fifth Edition: DSM-5.* (Arlington, VA: American Psychiatric Publishing, 2013); *and* The National Institute of Mental Health. See www.nimh.nih.gov/health/topics/eating-disorders/index.shtml (retrieved July 7, 2105).

11 American Psychiatric Association (2000) "Practice guidelines for treatment of patients with eating disorders (Revision)." *American Journal of Psychiatry*, 157 (1), 1–39.

12 David B. Herzog, Dara N. Greenwood, David J. Dorer, Andrea T. Flores, Elizabeth R. Ekeblad, Ana Richards, Mark A. Blais and Martin B. Keller (2000) "Mortality in eating disorders: A descriptive study." *International Journal of Eating Disorders*, 28, 20–26.

13 Pamela K. Keel and Tiffany A. Brown (2010) "Update on course and outcome in eating disorders." *International Journal of Eating Disorders*, 43 (3), 195–204. See also: Michael Strober, Roberta Freeman and Wendy Morrell (1997) "The long-term course of severe anorexia nervosa in adolescents: Survival analysis of recovery, relapse, and outcome predictors over 10–15 years in a prospective study." *International Journal of Eating Disorders*, 22 (4), 339–360.

14 Scott J. Crow, Carol B. Peterson, Sonja A. Swanson, Nancy C. Raymond, Sheila Specker, Elke D. Eckert and James E. Mitchell (2009) "Increased mortality in bulimia nervosa and other eating disorders." *American Journal of Psychiatry*, 166 (12), 1342–1346.

15 *Women, Food and God: An Unexpected Path to Almost Everything* (New York: Scribner, 2011) p. 37.

16 See www.orthorexia.com (retrieved July 7, 2105).

17 Barbara Mangweth-Matzek, Hans W. Hoek, Claudia I. Rupp, Kerstin Lackner-Seifert, Nadja Frey, Alexandra B. Whitworth, Harrison G. Pope and Johann Kinzl (2014) "Prevalence of eating disorders in middle-aged women." *International Journal of Eating Disorders*, 47, 320–324.

18 *Femininity* (New York: Linden Press/Simon & Schuster, 1984) p. 51.

19 American Psychiatric Association, op. cit., 300.7 (F45.22). See also David Porter, "Body Dysmorphic Disorder DSM-5 300.7 (F45.22)" at www. theravive.com/therapedia/Body-Dysmorphic-Disorder-DSM—5-300.7-(F45.22) (retrieved August 21, 2015).

20 Katharine A. Phillips, Sabine Wilhelm, Lorrin M. Koran, Elizabeth R. Didie, Brian A. Fallon, Jamie Feusner and Dan J. Stein (2010) "Body dysmorphic disorder: Some key issues for *DSM-V*." *Depression and Anxiety*, 27 (6), 573–591.

21 "Sign the beauty pledge." *O, The Oprah Magazine*, June, 2008. See www. oprah.com/spirit/Sign-the-Beauty-Pledge-O-Magazine-Beauty-Revolution-Pledge (retrieved September 11, 2015). Unfortunately, on October 19, 2015, Ms. Winfrey purchased a 10 percent ownership stake in Weight Watchers® and agreed to offer her name and face to no other weight-loss products for five years; see www.nytimes.com/2015/10/20/business/dealbook/shares-of-weight-watchers-jump-as-oprah-winfrey-takes-a-stake.html (retrieved October 30, 2015). Research shows that such programs contribute to yo-yo dieting. Even former Weight Watchers CFO Richard Samber admitted that the business was successful because the majority of customers regained the weight they lost, or as he put it: "That's where your business comes from." See Traci Mann, "Oprah's investment in Weight Watchers was smart because the program doesn't work" in *New York* Magazine, posted October 29, 2015, http://nymag. com/scienceofus/2015/10/why-weight-watchers-doesnt-work.html (retrieved October 30, 2015).

22 Katharine A. Phillips, William Menard and Christina Fay (2006) "Gender similarities and differences in 200 individuals with body dysmorphic disorder." *Comprehensive Psychiatry*, 47 (2), 77–87.

23 *Meditations for Women Who Do Too Much* (New York: HarperCollins, 1992) p. 27.

24 Margo Maine, *Body Wars: Making Peace with Women's Bodies* (Carlsbad, CA: Gürze Books, 2000).

25 See www.huffingtonpost.com/2015/04/21/woman-dies-diet-pills_n_7111518.html (retrieved July 1, 2015).

26 US Food and Drug Administration, "Beware of products promising miracle weight loss." See www.fda.gov/forconsumers/consumerupdates/ucm246742.htm (retrieved August 20, 2015).

27 Bruce D. Wadholtz, "Gastrointestinal complaints and function in patients with eating disorders." In Phillip S. Mehler and Arnold E. Anderson (Eds.) *Eating Disorders: A Guide to Medical Care and Complications* (Baltimore, MD: Johns Hopkins University Press, 1999) pp. 86–99.

28 For example, see www.spaindex.com/special-features/detox-retreats/ (retrieved July 7, 2105).

29 For instance, in 2014, the FDA issued 30 public notices and removed only seven weight loss products from the market. US Food and Drug Administration, op. cit.

30 Ibid.

31 ASPS Clearinghouse of Plastic Surgery Procedural Statistics (2014). "2013 Plastic Surgery Statistics Report" p. 6. See www.plasticsurgery.org/Documents/news-resources/statistics/2013-statistics/plastic-surgery-statistics-full-report-2013.pdf (retrieved July 2, 2015).

32 Ibid p. 20.

33 See www.statista.com/statistics/243742/revenue-of-the-cosmetic-industry-in-the-us/ (retrieved June 23, 2015).

34 *The Beauty Myth* (New York: William Morrow, 1991) p. 234.

35 ASPS (2014) op. cit.

36 See www.emandlo.com/2015/08/20-body-image-quotes-to-celebrate-national-underwear-day/. (retrieved September 11, 2015).

37 Katherine A. Phillips and Susan F. Diaz (1997) "Gender differences in body dysmorphic disorder." *Journal of Nervous and Mental Disease*, 185, 570–577.

38 Katharine A. Phillips, Jon Grant, Jason Siniscalchi and Ralph S. Albertini (2001). "Surgical and nonpsychiatric medical treatment of patients with body dysmorphic disorder." *Psychosomatics* 42, 504–510.

5   So Why Do People Do It?

> Understanding the difference between healthy striving and perfectionism is critical to laying down the shield and picking up your life. Research shows that perfectionism hampers success. In fact, it's often the path to depression, anxiety, addiction, and life paralysis.[1]
>
> Brené Brown

The symptoms of eating disorders are painful to contemplate. Just picture your child or best friend eating compulsively to fill her internal emptiness or sneaking off to the bathroom after every meal to purge. Or imagine that emptiness feels good, and emptier even better.

Imagine your partner or sister obsessively looking in every mirror she passes, compulsively changing clothes and leaving piles of discarded outfits behind, loading her suitcase with free weights when taking a weekend away, or running ten miles even though she has the flu. Imagine that she only feels good during the fleeting seconds after someone compliments her appearance.

Eating and body image obsessions isolate woman sufferers behind a thick wall of denial where they spend their energy looking inward, feeling frightened, despairing and alone. In this chapter, we'll explain that disordered eating and body image obsessions are not actually about eating, food, or weight. They are about the complex meanings that food, eating and body image assume when life seems frightening, empty and spinning out of control. They are about trying to be perfect in an imperfect world.

Who Has Them

For a long time, it appeared that only white, upper middle class and driven teenaged girls developed eating disorders and body image despair. That's not reality today, and probably never was. Instead, eating disorders and body image despair intrude upon the lives of women throughout all classes, races and ethnicities in our culture. They appear in girls as young as eight, geriatric patients and women of every age in between. A comprehensive research review finds no significant differences in body dissatisfaction between Caucasian, Hispanic and Asian women in the US.[2] For decades, Centers for Disease Control statistics on high risk dieting practices among adolescents have been compelling, and conclusively cross-cultural.

Decades ago, African-American women seemed unlikely to develop body image and eating problems because they lived in a matrilineal culture that honored women, and viewed strong, large female bodies as attractive. Self-worth grew primarily from spiritual strength, exemplified by and in big Black women.

But waves of multiculturalism (particularly multicultural marketing) brought widespread images of Black women with thin bodies and light skin—portrayed as most "attractive" when they move closest to the White ideal of beauty. Meanwhile, rapid cultural change (including pressure to "assimilate") loosened African-American women's ties to the protection of a strong, matrilineal heritage. This confluence of trends help explain the prevalence of eating and body image problems among African-American women.

Anorexia is the least frequent eating disorder in African-American and Caribbean-American women (as it also is for Caucasians), and binge eating disorder (BED) the most prevalent and persistent. Bulimia is more common among Black American women than previously believed,[3] probably due to multiple stressors including the stress of acculturation into a white dominant system.[4] Compelling books by Becky Thompson (*A Hunger So Wide and So Deep*[5]) and Stephanie Covington Armstrong (*Not All Black Girls Know How to Eat*[6]) poignantly describe the eating and body image struggles of African-American women. The myth that African-American women don't develop these problems is simply false.

The risk remains high for other women, including immigrants, trying to assimilate into the dominant definition of a successful woman: perfectly thin, perfectly groomed, perfectly sculpted and (usually) White. This exacerbates obsession about weight, food and appearance, which are already intense questions of identity for women trying to fit into our culture.

Meanwhile, women of color and less affluent social classes are unlikely to be referred to a physician or clinician to get help. Because outdated biases about who is at risk remain entrenched, health care professionals may overlook important signs of trouble and not even ask less affluent women about body image and eating concerns. Furthermore, the medical system has still not grasped the importance of screening for BED and other specified feeding or eating disorder (OSFED)—which affect women of all backgrounds. Such oversights keep sufferers from receiving appropriate diagnosis and lifesaving care.[7]

Fortunately, research indicates that Black women and girls who remain closely tied to family and community are more likely to reject media beauty ideals as unattainable—and not important in the opinions of family, friends and partners.[8] Instead, community-connected Black women and girls compare themselves to women they know, and judge beauty by standards of movement, character and style, rather than weight and appearance.

Eating disorders have become a universal language for women to convey difficult emotions and a deep sense of shame that they are not measuring up to today's standards for women. An eating disorder is the perfect answer to not being perfect in a culture that demands it.

Where They Are

> Thinness as a gendered body 'ideal' and a signifier of a multiplicity of positively construed 'attributes' can clearly no longer be considered exclusively western or white.[9]
>
> Mervat Nasser and Helen Malson

For many years, eating and body image concerns were found only in highly industrialized nations in North America and Western Europe. Globalization has changed this equation dramatically. Over 40 countries now report eating disorders prevalence, including Nigeria, India, China, South Korea, South Africa, former Soviet Republics and Mexico.[10] In one recent three-month period, the US-based National Eating Disorders Association hot line received calls from more than 70 different countries.[11]

As Western media saturate the globe, attitudes and behaviors about food and women's bodies shift markedly. A dramatic example occurred on the Pacific island of Fiji after US television arrived in 1995.

Long-held Fijian traditions valued large female bodies for their strength and contribution to family and community, while food was celebrated and enjoyed with deep ritual meaning. Similar traditions are common in less "developed" countries because eating is revered and celebrated in cultures where food tends to be scarce. A large body signifies that a woman has access to a most precious commodity: food. Big is her "shape of success," a sign of true well-being.

But globalized media can change this with blinding speed. After less than three years of limited exposure to mainstream US television fare, dieting and eating disorders—virtually non-existent before 1995—were rampant in Fiji. By 1998, 11 percent of Fijian women and girls engaged in self-induced vomiting, 29 percent were at risk for clinical eating disorders, 69 percent had dieted, and 74 percent felt "too fat."

Those three years brought no radical change in the Fijian diet or behavior (like an explosion in morbid obesity). The radical change came in the number of hours spent watching TV. Popular (and intensely marketed) female images on US television created a desire for Hollywood's super-thin "shape of success," quickly overturning centuries of strong Fijian traditions and values.[12]

Cross-cultural research indicates that eating and weight concerns may be higher in some Asian countries than in Western nations.[13] The increasing rates of eating disorders in Japan show the intersection of unhealthy beauty ideals with a culture that prioritize the needs and desires of a group over the individual's needs.[14]

The spread of Western media is not the only influence, however. With greater access to education, technologies, markets and paid employment worldwide, an unsettling process of transformation infuses women's personal lives. Meanwhile, powerful Western consumer culture infuses traditional local cultures, narrowing expectations about female appearance and beauty, dramatically revising the cultural role of women, and raising new questions about gender roles and gender justice. Like us, women in developing countries are becoming immigrants in their own land, as a new culture enters, making familiar surroundings suddenly seem foreign.

Global consumer culture also introduces the sedentary Western lifestyle and craftily marketed prepared foods, high in calories and fat. The resulting increase in obesity sparks self-defeating weight loss cycles—which creates demand for heavily marketed diet products and services. Along with swift shifts in cultural roles, global women and girls feel their learned reality about the female body colliding with Western body ideals in unfamiliar and dangerous ways.

Why They Are

Knowing the ethnicity and location of people with eating and body image obsessions doesn't tell us why some women start down such a destructive path, while others do not. Although we know many risk factors contributing to these multidimensional illnesses, we cannot predict who will and who will not develop the problem and what course the illness will take. I liken the onset of an eating disorder to a perfect storm: many elements have to be present, with the whole being much greater than the sum of its parts.

Research suggests that genetic, environmental and individual psychological factors all contribute.[15] Nature needs nurture. Women who grew up with an eating disorder sufferer in the family are more likely to fall victim themselves.[16] Women seem to have less chance of developing an eating disorder if they are resilient, manage stress well and use healthy coping skills—such as having postive body image, role models and support systems.

For women with eating disorders, however, the rituals of eating and body image obsessions initially provide a sense of comfort, control and security when dealing with life's transitions and stress. The rituals seem to work, and gradually become routine—but they risk our well-being and survival. Fixated on the shape we're in physically, the rest of our lives start unraveling.

Self-soothing

Women with eating disorders and body image despair use their compulsive eating, exercise, or appearance behavior to soothe their discomfort, stress, uncertainty, pain, sadness, desire and (eventually) all feelings. No matter where these women live, what color their skin, or how much money they have, these "self-soothing" rituals are central to their lives and identity.

So, how can anyone come to experience bingeing, vomiting, or starvation as self-soothing?

For women who binge or eat compulsively, the food temporarily fills up inner emptiness, distracts from distress, and/or numbs uncomfortable feelings. As with people who use alcohol or drugs to self-medicate, eating disorder patients often describe having a bottomless hole that they cannot fill.

For women with bulimia, vomiting and other purging provide physical (if temporary and dangerous) relief from pent-up emotional tension and stress, as well as a short-lived euphoric feeling due to brain chemistry changes which follow the purge.

When women with anorexia deny themselves food, they also get a short "high" (actually, dizziness due to chemical and nutritional imbalance). Exercise abusers may also feel temporarily invincible, at least until injuries and fatigue overpower the body's inherent limitations.

Even when sufferers understand the huge risks, most cannot stop on their own. The illusory sense of "being in control" feels irreplaceable while passing through times of intense emotion and substantial life changes. Operating under the distortion and delusion of the illness, they believe that nothing else will soothe their souls.

Many women who recovered from eating disorders report that their illness functioned, in a bizarre and destructive way, as a friend that provided feelings of stability and predictability. As one woman told me, "When everything else was changing, the eating disorder felt reliable, at least at first. It felt like it grounded me and was always there for me. But then it spun out of control, too."

Often, eating disorders emerge in response to physical and/or sexual abuse in our present or past. In fact, Post-Traumatic Stress Disorder (PTSD) is common among people with clinical eating disorders. A study of nearly 5,700 US adults found that the vast majority of women and men with anorexia, bulimia and BED "reported a history of interpersonal trauma. Rates of PTSD were significantly higher among women and men with BN and BED. Subthreshold PTSD was more prevalent than threshold PTSD among women with BN and women and men with BED."[17]

Starving, bingeing and other ritualistic eating disordered behaviors can symbolize limits to protect against further hurt or intrusion by abusers.[18] Purging can feel like a cathartic revulsion of the shameful, painful invasion of sexual trauma. Other times, the rituals manifest our (mistaken) belief that we don't deserve nourishment because we are dirty, worthless people who invited or deserved the abuse we endured.

Soon, the dangerous rituals numb and isolate us from any anger, anxiety and angst we feel about the trauma. People around us see these behaviors as self-punitive, continuing the pattern of pain. But the eating disordered abuse survivor perceives them as the most reliable way to care for herself. Her self-abuse feels more soothing than her trauma experiences. It briefly calms her, the way a sedative might.

In a sea of unresolved pain, the eating disorder feels like a life preserver we squeeze for dear life because we know no other way to swim to safety. Without alternate (healthy) ways to cope with life's waves, letting go of an eating disorder looks like a fatal mistake. But like life preservers, eating disorders offer only temporary relief. If a life preserver is our lone way to traverse the sea, we will surely drown. And since it keeps only one person afloat, we will surely drown alone.

Eating disorders and body image obsessions start out as self-soothing coping strategies that seem to help us through a difficult time or stage. But squeezing life into a scorecard of food, calories, pounds and clothing sizes reduces us to bouncing between brief spurts of feeling "soothed" and persisting periods of painful upheaval. Eating disorders and body image obsessions blind us to two crucial realities about soothing.

1. No problem can be solved with soothing alone. If we don't address, work through, and make peace with our problems, they keep resurfacing and we can't grow. As is true for everything else in nature, if we are not changing and growing, we are shrinking and dying.
2. We can be calmed in ways that don't destroy us, so we can learn healthy ways to self-soothe (see Chapter 9).

Control

Closely related to our desire to soothe life's discomforts is our desire to control them. The life transitions of ageing are disruptive, disorganizing and inevitable. Our culture glorifies the perfectly successful (and mythical) do-it-all Superwomen who seem unaffected by change and uncertainty. For many of us facing the prospect of unattainable perfection, micromanaging the shape of our bodies seems like a good substitute for setting our own standards and taking charge of our lives.

Our "image" may become as important as it was when we were 16. We fret over how other people see us as we pass through pregnancy, perimenopause, menopause and beyond—just like we did when we sprouted breasts, grew pubic hair and started menstruating. Rituals of not eating, overeating, purging and excess exercise look like ways to appear in control, when our inner lives feel chaotic.

Rachel, a 38-year-old married mother of three, was never encouraged to be an athlete as a girl. But after having children, she was drawn to jogging as a way to "manage her weight." She soon evolved from a recreational runner into an obsessively training marathoner. In addition to reducing her weight, running gave Rachel race-winning kudos that boosted her self-esteem while giving her a new identity and focus in her life. For a while, Rachel achieved racing goals that few other women her age could achieve.

Rachel used food and exercise rituals to gain a false sense of control over herself, how others saw her, and the many changes in her life. At least her weight was under control, even if everything else was changing with her kids growing up and her body starting to look and be older.

But Rachel's running remained compulsive and her weight dropped dangerously low. Soon, she developed knee problems and other injuries, because her undernourished body could no longer take the excessive exercise regimen. But Rachel wasn't listening to her body anymore and she kept on running despite the physical damage.

What brought Rachel into therapy, however, was worry over the negative comments that her teenage daughter was constantly making about her own body. In short order, Rachel and I were exploring her own anorexic behaviors. After resisting it for a long time, she gradually had to give up running because of her injuries.

However, she continued cutting her food intake more and more because, without the compulsive exercise, her body was taking longer to burn calories. Rachel developed elaborate and rigid rules about food, eating minimal amounts of low-fat food herself, while still cooking for her family, and trying to help her kids deal with their own adolescent body self-consciousness. After a year of therapy, Rachel still hadn't made peace with her changing body, her eating disorder, or her sense of self-loathing. She stopped coming to see me, and went back to struggling alone.

Some sufferers also say that their illness acted to "control" and repel invasive attention from strangers. As Mary put it, "Once my body became small, bony, frail, unattractive and androgynous-looking, then my body and I were much less likely to be sexually objectified by men and the culture. I really believed that my body shape was a radical political challenge to the objectification of women."

Other women say that weight gained after years of binge eating also acted as a "fat shield" to deflect unwanted sexualized attention. Kerry said: "I ate to create a buffer between me and the people who hurt me. My eating was disgusting, so I was disgusting. And I believed somehow that it would keep me safe."

Unfortunately, this fear of intrusion by objectification quickly slips into a compulsion to be untouchable. Erecting impenetrable walls erases hope of achieving connection, intimacy and true friendship. An initial attempt to protect oneself and/or make a powerful political statement ends up creating a place of empty powerlessness.

Identity

Over time, symptomatic behaviors become the core of the sufferer's identity. Women obsessed with body image and eating use their disorders to manufacture an identity that seems unique, memorable and worthy. On the surface, this seems to work. Cultural standards would have us believe that a woman who looks perfect *is* perfect—mastering every challenge that comes her way. The better looking our persona is, the better a person we are.

Starting in early childhood, external appearance and beauty pressures on girls create a lifelong link between our identity and our body. The link doesn't magically break as we age. Parameters for female achievement may have expanded, but female identity too often rests on the foundation of looks and sexual attractiveness.

For women with eating disorders, calories and weight obsession seem like a concrete strategy for obtaining internal and external advantages. After all, our culture and media glorify thin women, even those believed to be ill, urging us to emulate them. Body image and eating obsessions provide a script for crafting an "acceptable" image, which in turn defines our identity—even if the entire script is made of endless, rigid, perverse and destructive rules.

Gradually an inauthentic self emerges—one that *looks* happy, confident, and able to handle anything. But in reality, this false self has a flimsy and unsustainable foundation—based entirely on what we weigh, the size we wear, or how we look. Inside, we feel worse and worse as the eating disorder stifles our authentic self. Outside, our "public" shell grows more counterfeit and brittle, and we become afraid to drop the façade and admit reality.

Higher weight women with eating disorders struggle just as intensely as women emaciated by food restriction. Afraid of being found out, they feel tremendous pressure to hide their problems and to pretend they are happy. Many have dieted for decades without ever achieving the thin ideal. Any success they do achieve (academic accomplishment, raising a family, career, community leadership, or creative endeavors) is undermined by the shame of failing in their relationship with food and loathing of their bodies.

Many people with eating disorders panic when challenged to give up their rituals because they believe that their identity will disappear with it. Convinced that they will become invisible to themselves and others, they say things like these.

- But who will I be without my eating disorder?
- I am known as the one who doesn't eat. There is nothing else special about me.
- But I'm the skinny one; I'll disappear if I gain weight.
- This is my role in the family; the only thing anyone seems to notice. If I give it up, I'll be nothing again.
- What if I stop bingeing and still don't lose weight? I'll be an even bigger failure.

For many women in our culture—and, often, for the culture itself—body shape becomes indistinguishable from identity. We seem to live by the motto that "Bodies 'R' Us."

Beguiled by the "Benefits"

Like a very addictive drug, eating and body image compulsions are effective in the very short term. They briefly distract us from discomfort and/or numb pain.

But while a drug addict's haggard appearance seldom draws applause, a woman obsessed with body image can generate plenty of praise in our appearance-obsessed culture. Rigid adherence to our obsession may also provide fleeting feelings of superiority. Many sufferers find their outsides showered with complements ("You have such self-control! You look great!") while their insides are doubled over in pain, fear and shame. The praise is seductive, but simultaneously escalates the dissonance between body and spirit.

Other people's envy and adulation are difficult to give up. If we stop, everyone will know the real truth: we are imposters, not the "beautiful" persona we have portrayed. Medical providers echo the praise, making it even harder to let go of the behaviors.

But ultimately, the "power" of a polished look and sculpted body only increases our self-doubt—and the disorder's domination over us. As the gap between self-perception and other-perception widens, rituals of food, exercise and appearance become more central, and therefore more frightening to abandon.

It is appealing to judge ourselves and our world with the clarity of dichotomous standards: fat means failure and thin means success. But real life is more complex—and interesting—than arbitrary ideals of perfection that defy nature, eat away at our true identity, and are impossible to attain.

The Physical Process

> I'm in recovery from my bulimia for about as long as my husband
> has been sober from his alcoholism. There are many similarities
> between our situations, because my bulimia is very much like an
> addiction. But there's a very, very big difference, too.
>
> I know it's not always easy, but my husband can "put the plug
> in the jug" today without anywhere near the complications I face.
> Booze was a tiger that ripped apart his life, just like food and
> purging ripped apart my life. Thank God, we both learned ways to
> stay "sober" and lock each tiger up in a cage.
>
> But he won't starve if he never goes back to booze. I will starve
> if I never go back to food. I think of it like this: he can keep his
> tiger locked up, and choose not to think about today. I, on the other
> hand, have to take my tiger out of the cage for a walk three times
> a day.[19]
>
> Hannah

Unpleasant secondary physical symptoms also contribute to the
addictive hook of eating and body image disorders. For example, as
we fail to fuel our bodies with food, fatigue takes over and diet pills or
other stimulants may seem necessary to keep us awake and functioning.
The body easily becomes dependent on laxatives and withdrawal usually
results in painful constipation and weight gain due to fluid shifts (unless
detoxification is medically supervised). Similarly, withdrawal from
diuretics may generate unpleasant bloating or "water weight" because
the body instinctively holds onto extra fluid after being dehydrated.

Of course, eating disorder behaviors can quickly seem to make
unpleasant sensations of full and fat "go away," leaving us feeling empty
and in control again.

If we restrict food intake for substantial lengths of time, beginning
to eat sufficient food becomes a physical challenge for the body.
Responding to starvation cues, gastric secretions in the gut slow down.[20]
This keeps food in the stomach longer when we resume eating, making
us feel full and uncomfortable—and providing increased awareness of
that unwanted stomach.

> When I started eating again, every meal left me feeling like I did
> after a full Thanksgiving dinner in my childhood. I was absolutely
> stuffed even after eating very small amounts of food.[21]
>
> Melanie, a recovered adult

The physical changes of the illness and the discomfort of recovery
make it difficult to give up an eating disorder. Our health seems less
important than the symptom's short-term "rewards." The disorder's

destructive behaviors seem like foolproof methods for relieving pain and obtaining the ideal look that will (we hope!) lead to admiration and validation.

The Voice

Many women say the most powerful motivator for remaining on the deadly path of body and eating disorders is what they call "The Voice."

> I knew it was crazy to keep contributing to the physical problems that my anorexia brought down on me, or even to keep living with them. But that knowledge got drowned out by "The Voice." It felt like there was a mean little guy in my brain telling me that wrong was right, up was down, and that no matter what I did, I was fat, ugly and worthless and people didn't like me. Of course, people did like me—some even loved me—even when I was in the worst shape and having my worst days. But I never heard that. I felt like "The Voice" was leading me through a carnival fun house; all around me were mirrors that distorted every aspect of my life and who I am. Every day, I felt "The Voice" shouting lies in my ear, and I believed it.[22]
>
> Meredith

Even women without an eating disorder hear some version of "The Voice" trying to keep us "in our place" and distorting our ability to see and act on our strengths.

For eating disorders sufferers, "The Voice" feels deeply imbedded, drowning out the real voice and spirit of the authentic self. However, "The Voice" is not really a part of the sufferer. It is part of the *illness* and separate from the person's identity. The language of fat and body image despair is very potent throughout our culture.

To help distinguish the voice from the self, I sometimes encourage patients to externalize it and call it a name like "ED" (short for Eating Disorder) as a reminder that "The Voice" is not their own voice.[23]

"The Voice," "ED," or whatever we call it, keeps sufferers on a short leash, always yanking their chain, leaving them uncertain of their own convictions. In fact, "The Voice" gains power by making sufferers feel like they can't survive or succeed without their disorder.[24]

Detecting "The Voice"

Take a look at the chart overleaf. How many of the following statements do you hear in your head? How often? Be honest with your responses; no one will judge you on your answers.

	Never	Weekly	Daily	Multiple times a day
You are a failure.				
You are ugly and eating makes you uglier.				
You are fat and disgusting.				
Food is evil, and will make you fat.				
You don't deserve anything.				
No one really cares about you.				
If you eat, you'll get fat and people will like you even less.				
Only weak people eat.				
You are a big disappointment.				
You are worthless.				
You deserve to feel lousy.				
Your body is repulsive.				
You are strong only when you don't eat / when you purge / when you exercise.				
No one is ever going to want to be with you if they find out who you really are.				

The thoughts in this list control us by attacking our self-esteem, degrading us and convincing us to ignore and deny the damage they cause. Whether or not you have an eating disorder, keep track of how often these thoughts intrude. Recognize them, challenge them, and share them in therapy. They gradually will become less powerful and convincing, but this will take time and practice. "The Voice" is stubborn and doesn't give up easily.

"The Voice" doesn't have an on-off switch. Most of us hear it a little bit and face the challenge of turning down its volume and developing a more positive, alternative voice to counteract it. "The Voice" seldom disappears entirely, but eating and body image recovery starts when a sufferer decides to quiet and manage the voice, and listen to it less.

Even now, years past anorexia, that sense of an independent force persists, as though some judgmental entity—me, but not quite me— lives on in a corner of my mind where it stands watch, always aware of the body, attuned to every nuance of shape and heft and contour, always anticipating the worst, always poised to deliver a slap at any hint of laziness or sloth or relaxed control. Sometimes the voice is proactive: Don't eat that brownie, don't take seconds; you'll feel pious, you'll feel resolute and thin. More often, it's punitive, a voice of sneering disdain: Look at that stomach. Look at those thighs. You're turning into a cow.[25]

Caroline Knapp

"The Voice" thought process capitalizes on the seduction of the positives, reinforcing illusions of control. Psychologists call this dichotomous reasoning: a tendency to see things only in the extremes, such as saintliness vs. evil or success vs. failure. We come to see ourselves as all one or all the other—moral or worthless, thin or fat—but unable to see any nuance in-between.

This is an unforgiving way to live. This rigid system of impossible expectation and self-perception defies the rich and beautiful imperfections of real life and real people. It magnifies endless self-defeating messages of failure and inadequacy which, in turn, continue fueling the obsessions with weight, food and body image.

Gradual Adaptation

Over time, persistent habits begin to feel normal, whether or not they are good for us. We just get used to doing what we do and feeling what we feel, even if those actions and emotions are deadly. With eating disorders, sensations as essential and basic as hunger and fullness become so completely masked that sufferers have no idea whether they are hungry, full or somewhere in between.

Any food in the stomach feels uncomfortable and yet the stomach growls and gurgles. Do those sensations mean the body wants more or is it complaining of too much? Women with eating disorders have lost their capacity to know the answer, because the malnourished brain can no longer decipher signals sent from the digestive system.

That's why it is useless to tell a sufferer "just eat til you feel full" or "listen to your hunger." It takes a lot of nutrition and practice to reclaim knowledge of these very basic states. Experienced dietitians and therapists often prescribe a meal plan focused on fueling the body at regular intervals with sufficient nutrients as a first step to re-teaching the body how to decode hunger and fullness cues. It takes time, patience and guts to reclaim this basic body knowledge. (There is more on the recovery process in Chapters 9 and 10.)

Surprisingly, it is easy to get used to feeling physically lousy. We can adapt to virtually anything if it creeps up on us slowly, as eating disorders do. Vitality, concentration and mood gradually deteriorate during the illness. Incrementally, we feel less energetic, less in tune with what is happening around us, and less able to focus and think things through. The slow pace of change can blind families and friends to the problem; they may not pick up signs that an outsider might. Meanwhile, the sufferer completely loses track of how she used to feel.

Soon, falling asleep on the job or while driving may become normal for a woman with an eating disorder. She may wake up in the middle of the night and binge because her body is literally trying to keep her alive. But even those incidents may not be visible to others because a woman with an eating disorder dedicates great energy to covering up her fatigue, malaise and muddled thinking. She works harder and harder at keeping up appearances, and this increased effort eventually feels normal as well. The disorder's demands, combined with the volume of "The Voice," make it nearly impossible to tune into her inner state or to hear the concern of loved ones. She is genuinely unaware that she's running on empty.

Vomiting, laxatives, diet pills, starving, bingeing, or excess-exercise are all unusual, unpleasant things to do. But as "The Voice" brainwashes, eating disorder behaviors also appear normal after a while. Strange and destructive habits soon become central to our identity as they temporarily tame relentless negative self-perceptions and emotions.

Gradually, the eating disorder becomes a precious cloak. Even as it morphs into a steadily tightening straightjacket, the cloak of disease feels so comfortable, so safe, something no one can take away. What began as a relief from life's problems takes on a life of its own. The destructive habits and negative self-talk are so ingrained that we use them even when we don't really feel so bad. Eventually we automatically and mindlessly do self-destructive behaviors every time we think we won't be caught.

> It was in my 40s, and if you suffer from bulimia, the older you get, the worse it gets. It takes longer to recover from a bout. I had to make a choice: I live or I die.[26]
>
> Jane Fonda

Denial

A cornerstone of any eating disorder is a sufferer's denial of its existence, seriousness and full implications. As with addiction to alcohol or heroin, denial serves as a stubborn barrier between illness and recovery.

Eating disorders contribute to denial because malnutrition starves the brain, clouding insight and awareness of the problem. (The technical term for the inability or refusal to recognize a physical or mental condition is anosognosia, which occurs across a variety of medical and psychiatric disorders.) Since malnutrition is a problem in binge eating, anorexia and bulimia, nutritional rehabilitation is essential to feed that starving brain and give it the capacity to work toward recovery.

Gradual adaptation helps denial to blossom: once we've gotten used to bingeing, purging, or starving, we believe that there is nothing abnormal about these behaviors, completely losing touch with the body's cues. Like an alcoholic who spends hours in bars, we may surround ourselves with people who share our symptoms, building up denial's ability to normalize sick conduct. Or, like the alcoholic who drinks alone at home, we may just keep our symptoms so secret that we do not admit or "see" them.

But denial has even more cunning, baffling and powerful qualities.

When confronted by unavoidable facts, many adult women with eating disorders refuse to believe the illness' impact on the body. Even when the body begins to have heart abnormalities, diabetes, osteoporosis, bloody stools and vomit—denial can refuse to budge.

These women revisit the adolescent state of omnipotence, convinced that they are somehow immune from the devastating results of an eating disorder. In therapy, they tell me:

- That won't happen to me; I'm different.
- Those rules apply to everyone else; I'm okay doing this.
- This damage isn't because of my eating.
- Don't worry; I'm in control. I know just what I can do and get away with.
- I'm not really sick; I don't weigh 75 pounds and I've never had to be forcefed through a tube.

Steeped in denial, women with eating disorders stubbornly ignore the signals and second chances their bodies provide. If the denial doesn't break down, their bodies eventually will. Permanent, irreversible damage happens. Second chances expire and suicide, choking, bleeding of the esophagus, cardiac arrest, or other organ failures eventually can (and do) kill.

Frequently, the physical damage resulting from eating disorders isn't visible until a medical crisis occurs. Laboratory tests and blood work can be normal one hour and deadly the next. The physical day of reckoning often comes too late. That is why it is so important to demolish denial before the eating disorder demolishes life itself.

The Doctor's Perspective

Health care professionals continue to overlook how frequently eating disorders and body image despair affect adult women. Much of the medical community still believes these are adolescent issues, making it hard for adult women to get appropriate help.

Furthermore, health care biases sometimes foster the problem instead of confronting it. Remember the story of Jennifer from Chapter 1. Desperate for help, she finally felt ready to confide in her physician, only to hear him and his staff praise her weight loss. They never even asked how she achieved it or how she felt about it. Demoralized and discouraged by the doctor's remarks, Jennifer left his office more disoriented and alone than when she entered. Fortunately, she did not give up and eventually found recovery resources. Wisely, she also found a new physician.

Medicine and health care have made major advances in recent years, many of them beneficial to women. But there remain cultural and financial forces in medicine that still wage war on our bodies. For example, standards designed to determine healthy or "ideal" weights rely on narrow, simplistic formulas. Since weight is easy and cheap to track, insurance companies began collating weight with mortality, even though there is seldom a direct connection between the two.

The original standards, published by New York Metropolitan Life Insurance Company in the 1940s (revised several times since), equated *average* weight with *ideal* weight. They also allowed no adjustment for age (even though men and women gain natural and healthy weight at different ages), increased insurance premiums for people who added pounds during adulthood, and fostered the false impression that weight was the country's primary health problem.[27]

Met Life's tables and the more recent Body Mass Index (BMI) formula retain outsized influence. Health care professionals continue to misperceive the connection between weight and health. Capitalizing on these flaws, the diet industry is a profiteer's dream come true, with a self-generating market renewed by the industry's own inherent failure rate. Even children feel the effects.

- Forty-two percent of girls in grades 1 through 3 want to lose weight.[28]
- Forty-five percent of children in grades 3 through 6 want to be thinner; 37 percent have already been on a diet.[29]
- Half of 9- and 10-year-old girls feel better about themselves when dieting.[30]
- Nine percent of 9-year-old girls say they have vomited to lose weight.[31]
- Girls say they are more afraid of being fat than of a parent dying.
- By high school, 70 percent of normal weight girls feel fat and go on diets.[32]

Medical personnel indoctrinated in the war against obesity tend to idealize all forms of weight loss instead of examining the reasons and methods behind them. In fact, how we lose weight is usually more important than how much weight we lose. When medical providers encourage overly restrictive eating or overemphasize weight as the prime indicator of health, they can trigger bingeing (in response to deprivation and hunger), exercise abuse, severe food restriction, body loathing and purging—even in women who never before obsessed about food and body image. Focusing merely on weight without asking other relevant questions, too many physicians ignore essential clues to the nature of women's relationship to food, body and health.[33]

The brief, pressured face-to-face doctor consultations of our managed care medical system raise additional barriers. Women already sensitive to being judged or misunderstood come away from rushed exams and curt comments feeling that their concerns and symptoms don't really merit attention or treatment. Excruciating embarrassment and shame result from being weighed in an open area (as many clinics do) or hearing insensitive comments and jokes around the scale. When starting treatment, some of my adult patients admit that they haven't seen a doctor in years, because such experiences were so painful.

Adult women struggling with body image and eating disorders desperately need medical resources, but too few traditionally trained health care professionals know how to provide informed and appropriate care. I spend many hours preparing clients for their medical visits and decoding the mixed messages doctors and nurses give.

To be fair, the medical profession reflects the biases of the larger culture in which they and we live. To help address the problem, I developed a simple list of questions to screen adult women at routine medical appointments. This can start a much needed dialogue about women, weight and the medical profession's role in keeping a woman free from an eating disorder. The questions don't take long and could help to identify people who physicians can refer for appropriate treatment.

- Has your weight fluctuated during your adult years?
- Are you trying to "manage" your weight?
- If so, how?
- What did you eat yesterday?
- How much do you think or worry about weight, shape and food?[34]

I also train medical professionals on the impact of insensitive comments and how to assess and intervene with eating disorders and body image despair. But far more initiative must come from within the medical establishment. It is truly heart-breaking when medical treatment is part of the problem rather than the solution.

The Physicians' Role in the Prevention of Eating Disorders

Primary prevention: Reducing or eliminating the problem by understanding and addressing causes and risk factors. Physicians are doing primary prevention whether they know it or not when they:

- educate patients about nutrition
- play the role of health educator
- encourage healthy physical activity

- promote positive body image
- help families to communicate effectively, have healthy relationships, and build self-esteem
- guide parents and children through the challenges of growth and individuation
- discuss the natural changes in a woman's body as she ages, including a lower metabolic rate and likely weight gain around menopause.

Secondary prevention: Identifying the problem early, before it becomes severe. Physicians play an important role by:

- noticing changes in physical parameters such as growth, weight and vital signs
- sharing concerns and providing initial counseling
- educating patients about the importance of adequate nutrition and health habits
- consulting with schools, athletic organizations and other influential groups
- sharing information about eating disorders in adults, and in people of color.

Tertiary prevention: Developing strategies to keep the problem from getting worse. Physicians are unique in their ability to:

- refer for appropriate therapy by knowing the resources in their area
- break the denial by giving an historic perspective of their observations of the patient's condition and potential consequences of the eating disorders
- educate patients about the positive benefits of treatment
- monitor the medical status and keep patients stable while treatment proceeds
- set a positive example of needing others by collaborating and communicating with mental health professionals
- advocate for appropriate care when insurance denies it.

Notes

1 *The Gifts of Imperfection: Let Go of Who You Think You're Supposed to Be and Embrace Who You Are* (Center City, MN: Hazelden, 2010) p. 56.
2 Shelly Grabe and Janet Shibley Hyde (2006). "Ethnicity and body dissatisfaction among women in the United States: A meta-analysis." *Psychological Bulletin*, 132, 622–640.

3 Jacquelyn Y. Taylor, Cleopatra Howard Caldwell, Raymond E. Baser, Nakesha Faison and James S. Jackson (2007) "Prevalence of eating disorders among blacks in the National Survey of American Life." *International Journal of Eating Disorders*, 40, S10–S14.

4 Marisol Perez, Zachary R. Voelz, Jeremy W. Petit and Thomas E. Joiner (2002). "The role of acculturative stress and body dissatisfaction in predicting bulimic symptomatology across ethnic groups." *International Journal of Eating Disorders*, 31, 442–454.

5 Minneapolis, MN: University of Minnesota Press, 1996.

6 Chicago, IL: Chicago Review Press, 2009.

7 Fary M. Cachelin and Ruth H. Striegel-Moore. (2006) "Help seeking and barriers to treatment in a community sample of Mexican American and European American women with eating disorders." *International Journal of Eating Disorders*, 39, 154–161.

8 Deborah Schooler, L. Monique Ward, Ann Merriwether and Allison Caruthers (2004) "Who's that girl: Television's role in the body image development of young white and black women." *Psychology of Women Quarterly*, 28 (1), 40.

9 "Beyond western dis/orders: Thinness and self-starvation of other-ED women." In Helen Malson and Maree Burns (Eds.) *Critical Feminist Approaches to Eating Dis/orders* (London: Routledge, 2009) pp. 74–86.

10 Richard Gordon "Eating disorders East and West: A culture-bound syndrome unbound." In Mervat Nasser, Melanie A. Katzman and Richard A. Gordon (Eds.) *Eating Disorders and Cultures in Transition* (London: Brunner-Routledge, 2001) pp. 1–16.

11 Personal communication with Margo Maine.

12 Anne E. Becker, Rebecca A. Burwell, David B. Herzog, Paul Hamburg and Stephen E. Gilman (2002) "Eating behaviours and attitudes following prolonged exposure to television among ethnic Fijian adolescent girls." *The British Journal of Psychiatry*, 180 (6), 509–514.

13 Jane Wardle, Anne M. Haase and Andrew Steptoe (2006) "Body image and weight control in young adults: International comparisons in university students from 33 countries." *International Journal of Obesity*, 30, 644–651.

14 Mihoko Kusano-Schwarz and Jörn von Wietersheim (2005) "EDI results of Japanese and German women and possible sociocultural explanations." *European Eating Disorders Review*, 13, 411–416.

15 Kristen M. Culbert, Sarah E. Racine and Kelly L. Klump (2015) "Research review: What we have learned about the causes of eating disorders—a synthesis of sociocultural, psychological, and biological research." *Journal of Child Psychology and Psychiatry*. In press. doi: 10.1111/jcpp.12441.

16 Richard Rende "Liability to psychopathology: A quantitative genetic study." In Linda Smolak, Michael P. Levine and Ruth H. Striegel-Moore (Eds.) *The Developmental Psychopathology of Eating Disorders: Implications for Research, Prevention and Treatment.* (Mahwah, NJ: Lawrence Erlebaum Associates, 1996) pp. 59–76.

17 Karen S. Mitchell, Suzanne E. Mazzeo, Michelle R. Schlesinger, Timothy D. Brewerton and Brian N. Smith (2012) "Comorbidity of partial and subthreshold PTSD among men and women with eating disorders in the national comorbidity survey-replication study." *International Journal of Eating Disorders*, 45 (3), 307–315.

18 See David Emerson, "Yoga as an adjunctive treatment for posttraumatic stress disorder." In Carolyn Costin and Joe Kelly (Eds.) *Yoga and Eating Disorders: Ancient Healing for a Modern Illness* (New York: Routledge, 2016) pp. 43–52.

19 Personal communication with Joe Kelly, 2001.

20 Bruce D. Wadholtz, "Gastrointestinal complaints and function in patients with eating disorders." In Phillip S. Mehler and Arnold E. Anderson (Eds.) *Eating Disorders: A Guide to Medical Care and Complications.* (Baltimore, MD: Johns Hopkins University Press, 1999) pp. 86–99.
21 Personal communication with Margo Maine.
22 Personal communication with Margo Maine.
23 Many people appreciate Jenni Shafer's books, *Life Without Ed* (New York: McGraw-Hill Education, 2003) and *Good Bye Ed. Hello Me* (New York: McGraw-Hill Education, 2009) for their examples of how externalizing the disorder can help a sufferer to regain her sense of self and recover.
24 For an illustration of this phenomenon, see Dina Zeckhausen and Bryan Mercer's musical play *What's Eating Katie?* See www.whatseatingkatie.com/ (retrieved September 22, 2015).
25 *Appetites: Why Women Want* (Berkeley, CA: Counterpoint Press, 2011) p. 63.
26 Laura Brown, "Jane Fonda: The interview." *Harper's Bazaar*, August, 2011. See www.harpersbazaar.com/celebrity/latest/news/a769/jane-fonda-interview/ (retrieved November 12, 2015).
27 Glenn A. Gasser, *Big Fat Lies: The Truth about Your Weight and Your Health* (Carlsbad, CA: Gürze Books, 2002).
28 M. Elizabeth Collins. (1991). "Body figure perceptions and preferences among preadolescent children." *International Journal of Eating Disorders*, 10, 199–208.
29 Michael J. Maloney, Julie McGuire, Stephen R. Daniels and Bonny Specker (1989) "Dieting behavior and eating attitudes in children." *Pediatrics*, 84 (3) 482–489.
30 Laurel M. Mellin, Charles E. Irwin Jr. and Sarah Scully (1992) "Prevalence of disordered eating in girls: A survey of middle-class children." *Journal of the American Dietetic Association*, 92 (7), 851–853.
31 Ibid.
32 Christine Ferron (1997) "Body image in adolescence in cross-cultural research." *Adolescence*, 32, 735–745.
33 An excellent resource explaining the medical issues and assessment process is Edward P. Tyson, "Medical assessment of eating disorders." In Margo Maine, Beth Hartman McGilley and Douglas Bunnell (Eds.), *Treatment of Eating Disorders: Bridging the Research–Practice Gap.* (London: Elsevier, 2010) pp. 89–110.
34 Margo Maine, "The weight-bearing years: Eating disorders and body image despair in adult women." Ibid., pp. 285–300.

6   How Family Shapes Us

> While you can take the woman out of the kitchen, can you really take
> the kitchen out of the woman?[1]
>
> Jane Rachel Kaplan

At 38 years old, Joan sought me for therapy because she worried about
her reactions to her children's eating. She sometimes pushed food on the
kids, but then was afraid that they were eating too much. To counter the
fear, Joan restricted their snacks, making sure that only perfectly "good"
food was in the house. She was terrified that her children, especially her
six-year-old daughter, might end up fat.

Joan soon acknowledged her own bulimia, while insisting that her
children not learn about it. She saw her eating disorder as a personal
moral failure and felt defective—like an "out-of-control freak." Joan acted
as her own prosecutor, judge and jury—indicting, blaming and shaming
herself. She also desperately wanted to be sure her children didn't end up
with painful eating disorders.

When I asked about her own childhood, Joan described her father as
far more dedicated to work than to his family. When he was around, he
tended to be critical and harsh. Joan's mother and other family members
rarely stood up to her father because he was easily angered and not so
easily calmed. Joan blamed herself for causing his rage and disrupting
the family peace. While her father routinely pressured Joan to eat large
quantities of food, she also knew that he valued thinness, especially in
women. She worried that eating might please him in the short term, but
that a fat body would anger him in the long term. By her early teens, Joan
found a secret way to avoid this dilemma—she started to purge.

Initially, Joan resisted talking about her parents during therapy,
defensively asking why her family history mattered. Grudgingly, she
traced the lasting impacts of her father's intrusive demands about food
and appearance and she understood how her symptoms helped her
cope. Bulimia made Joan feel like she exerted control over her weight by
vomiting, while pleasing her father by eating.

For years Joan believed she had no choice over either her food intake or the expectation that she should be thin. She *had* to eat what people offered, just as she had to eat for her father. She *had* to be thin and look good for others, especially her father. During therapy, however, Joan recognized that her father needed to control and choreograph everything around him, not just her. Appreciating the link between her decades of bulimia and the excessive power her father exerted, she discovered a larger family context in which her bulimia made sense.

Joan didn't talk to her father about her new insights because she wanted to avoid being disappointed by his response. Nevertheless, she also began to connect the dots between *his* childhood and his attitude about food during *her* childhood. As a boy, Joan's father had to help raise his siblings after his own father died. Money and food were scarce and he began working when he was a child to help support his family. Because of these experiences, food was never a neutral substance to Joan's father. Food's symbolism in his life made eating both a privilege and a duty.

As her treatment progressed, Joan admitted how angry she was at her mother for not asserting more strength in her marriage. Joan felt conflicted about this anger because she also knew that her mom sacrificed much of her own life for the family. She began to grasp that her mother never openly endorsed female appetites or ambitions (including her own or Joan's). With this insight, Joan discovered how unprepared she was for the complexities of being a woman today.

In learning about the dynamics between Dad, Mom, siblings and herself, Joan became more aware and comfortable handling food and dealing with interactions surrounding eating with her own children and husband. Joan still struggled to trust her children's appetites, but with help, she began to separate her food issues from theirs. Like many mothers with eating disorders, Joan needed a great deal of support on this because she was still primarily responsible for feeding the family. The children were her initial motivation for seeking treatment, and she didn't want to disappoint them.

Joan's husband, Steve, was a warm, loving man but had little understanding of Joan's illness or the stress she felt as a daughter and a parent. He wasn't particularly intuitive or inquisitive and sometimes thought that problems were best handled by being left alone. Compared to his contemporaries, Steve was an involved dad, but he duplicated his own parents' example and left most childrearing decisions up to Joan.

Joan's increasing ability to assert herself in her marriage was an important step in her treatment. Eventually she involved Steve in therapy sessions to help address their partnership and communication issues. Steve responded with the willingness to change, and he became a more active and supportive husband and father. This strengthened their marriage and took some pressure off Joan. She was especially happy when they both felt freer to develop their own personal parenting styles, independent of the previous generation's dynamics.

Despite all of her progress, Joan still resisted giving up her destructive coping behaviors. After decades of inconsistent eating and purging, it was hard to stop defining her feelings through her body and judging her self-worth by bulimia's distorted standard. Gradually, Joan tolerated her discomfort with how more normal eating might affect her appearance. Joan did gain weight, while therapy helped her to see many other things she gained as well—valuable things that bulimia always denied her.

> Experiencing our beauty as ever-changing works of art is an essential ingredient to living a life of freedom and meaning—and helping our children do the same.[2]
>
> Connie Sobczak

Still, after 25 years with an eating disorder, Joan's first impulse when angry, upset, or anxious is to purge or restrict her eating. Like many women in recovery, she occasionally returns to her symptoms. She is not perfect, but she works on understanding the contributing stressors and no longer indicts herself when she slips. She is steadily developing other coping mechanisms to replace her eating disorder. Joan feels like she can be more herself and feels her self-worth growing. She now believes that her wants, needs and hungers are acceptable and should be met. Just as she has come to understand the multiple reasons for her father's behavior, she is also learning to connect the dots about the effects of her own. And she can forgive both her family and herself.

The Family Table

While we can never fully decipher the mystery that is family, our best classroom may be the dinner table. Food is never just a neutral tool for nutrition; all families and cultures fill food with symbolism, meaning and emotion. That's why anthropologists turn to food customs and rituals to understand a culture's social structure, social values, celebratory rituals and communication methods. A culture's food related rituals both reveal and reinforce mores about power, gender, roles, class, social order and belief systems.

Historically, women's cultural role has been closely tied to providing and preparing food for others, especially our families. Usually, we begin food-related chores as girls—setting the table, cleaning up, serving others—before taking on primary responsibility as adults for shopping and cooking. Our food-related roles also teach us to nurture others but not always ourselves. Food is always around us, and for most women, it is an inescapable part of our identity, often in positive ways. Yet at the same time, food is a potential enemy, threatening to make us feel fat and imperfect if we dare to indulge our appetites.

Ethnicity and heritage also influence our relationships to food. For example, many immigrant families retain their traditional food choices, preparation and customs to feel a sense of continuity during the transition to a new culture. Even if our clan has lived here for centuries, we still use ethnic foods to celebrate family occasions: corned beef and cabbage; grits and fatback; pasta and meatballs; bratwurst and kraut; kung pao chicken. Despite this rich and lasting heritage, we seldom (if ever) talk about the multiple meanings food has in our families and lives. Few of us conceptualize how much our relationship to food is our own, and how much is dictated by family, history, ancestors and culture.

Perfect Eaters

When we look at our family of origin as an anthropologist would, we learn interesting things. Consider the perfectionistic clean plate club that some parents impose on their children. It often reflects the family and cultural experience (e.g., where food was very tightly controlled or scarce) which our parents and grandparents brought from their childhood to our first dining table. Other parents insist that children eat specific foods (whether they like them or not), eat according to a very rigid schedule, or eat constantly regardless of hunger.

Clearly, parents don't raise "perfect eaters" with malicious intent, in order to teach an abstract moral lesson, or because their eating will do anything to help today's starving children. They do it because of the things food symbolizes for them. Nevertheless, pressure on a child to please parents by eating can easily confuse her ability to assess and respond to her basic hunger and satiety. Guilt for wanting more can trigger restricting and fear of deprivation can spark compulsive eating. Some children eventually purge to take some control over how the "perfect eater" ethic affects their lives.

Of course, some women from families of "perfect eaters," addiction, abuse and other problems respond with balanced, healthy attitudes and behaviors about eating, emotion and food. Why do some of us grow up with disturbed notions about food and eating while others of us grow up with devil-may-care attitudes? There is no easy answer based on the scientific and psychosocial knowledge we have today. The emotional health and socioeconomic status of our family are factors. Genetics play a role, although we still know precious little about their influence. Many factors come together in a perfect biopsychosocial storm to result in an eating disorder.

Eating Lessons

Look at these questions and take some time to think about the lessons your families taught about eating.

- What were my family's unspoken rules about food and eating?
- What happened if I challenged or broke these rules?
- How was food tied into other family dynamics, like rewarding and punishing behavior (mine or someone else's)?
- Who was in charge of my eating?
- How important were my own cues or desires? Were they respected?
- How did my family's eating patterns relate to our ethnic or cultural background?
- What was my mother's relationship to food? My father's? My siblings'? My grandmother's? My grandfather's? Other important people in my family?
- How has my eating been affected by theirs?
- What were the lessons I learned about food? Was it something to be enjoyed, feared, cherished, or hated?
- What emotions were tied to food and eating?
- Have I passed on any of these lessons and feelings to others?
- Is there anything I need or want to change about myself in light of these patterns?

Answering these questions will help us to understand our present situations, and if we are a parent, can help us avoid repeating negative patterns.

The Family-Built Body Image

In many ways, our personal and idiosyncratic body image is a shared body image, crafted in part by both family and culture. Even before birth, expectant parents and grandparents imagine how their babies will look and anticipate their body characteristics or abilities ("He'll have the build for football" or "I want her to be a ballerina"). When we see a newborn in her crib, we form body associations—"She looks just like Aunt Susie"— that also have emotional associations, depending on how we feel about Aunt Susie.

It is natural for parents and family members to be pleased by certain characteristics of our bodies and appearance, and this can be a good thing. However, most girls also feel a conflict between extremes, sensing that a boyish, athletic body may satisfy Dad, while more feminine characteristics may please Mom, or vice versa.

Much of our response is unconscious, layering our family's perceptions of our body atop our own developing sense of body. If our family places a high value on external beauty, we may gain some degree of acceptance and approval by living up to the standard—even if it means sacrificing our ability to know and love our natural bodies. Or we may rebel against the look that we know will please our families, just to assert some authority in our lives. Either way, our bodies take on importance.

As our bodies change during adolescence, the family investment in our body image remains. Perhaps we tried to keep our bodies small, young and less mature in an attempt to avoid the challenges of growing up, delay the loss of childhood security and remain close to a parent:

> My father and I were very close and affectionate. But as soon as I started developing breasts, he stopped hugging me. I instinctively knew that that was why. I decided that if my breasts were going to get in the way, I'd try to make them stop—and try to make myself stop growing up—because I didn't want to lose him. So I stopped eating. And I ended up in the hospital with anorexia.[3]

Some of my adult patients struggle to accept themselves because, well into adulthood, their families retain a deep and ongoing stake in the culture's unnaturally perfectionistic ideals for beauty and weight. For them, self-improvement means doing just about anything to change their bodies in pursuit of family approval.

Of course many of our mothers, grandmothers and other family matriarchs "did" aging in positive ways. But we may not have confidence that the lessons of their lives apply to ours. That can leave us feeling out of sync with our nearest role models, uncertain of what will happen next, ambivalent about our bodies, and willing to abuse them.

Step Back Exercise II

Do this alone, with a friend, or in a small group of women you trust, building in time to talk about your feelings and insights afterward.

- Stand comfortably, preferably without shoes, so you can feel the ground or floor. Keep enough space around you to be able to move back and forward several feet.
- Close your eyes and relax.
- Take a step backward and imagine that you are stepping into your body of ten years ago. Take a few minutes to get used to

being in this body and mind-set. Remember how your body felt and what it meant to you.

- Take another step backward and step into your body of twenty years ago. Take a few minutes to reacquaint yourself with how it feels to be in this body and mindset.
- Continue this routine, one decade at a time, until you reach your early twenties. With each step back, take time to get used to being in that life and body.
- Next, step back to your high school body. Again soak up what this body feels and means to you.
- Continue to roll back the clock by stepping into your body in elementary school, then as a preschooler, and then your body in your earliest memories.
- Finally, step back a bit further and imagine what your infant and toddler body felt like.
- Stay in that baby body and imagine how your family responded to your shape, your weight, your appearance and your appetite.
  - Did they like how you looked as a baby?
  - Did you feel criticized or accepted; what was your body esteem?
  - Did your family think you were eating too much or not enough?
- Now step forward to being a toddler and ask those same questions.
- Step forward to preschool and then elementary school, asking the same questions.
- Now step forward to your adolescent body and remember how your family responded to you.
- Step forward to your late teens and early twenties, asking again what messages your family was giving you about your body, weight, appetites.
- Step forward a decade at a time to the present, considering what messages you received from your family. Are they different now than they were then?

Reflecting on this exercise, can you identify family messages that were harmful to your body image and sense of self? Can you identify family messages that were positive? Were there any particular turning points in your body image and feelings about your needs and appetites?

Take a few minutes to absorb these insights. How did body or beauty concerns evolve throughout these years? In what ways do you feel connected to your family's messages? In what ways do you feel alone or disconnected from your family or from your past?

What surprised you as you traversed these bodies and eras in your life? How do you feel about this experience?

Write these perceptions down in a journal so you can reflect on them over time. If you do the exercise in a group, make time to share your experiences and insights with one another.

Family Dynamics

You can observe a lot just by watching.[4]

Yogi Berra

In Louise's family, everyone had to be happy and nice to one another. Conflict, anger, anxiety and tension weren't allowed out in the open, even after Louise's grandmother moved in and strained everyone's established routine. Because the emotional electricity was never discharged, Louise developed no skills or experience in expressing difficult emotions.

Nevertheless, Louise did sense that she *had* lots of those feelings. However, since there were no signs that anyone else in the family shared them, Louise felt different and alone. She felt sure that the others must be right and she was wrong.

As a teen, Louise felt lucky that her body included features fitting the culture's (and her family's) beauty standard. She came to feel that her appearance was her most important attribute. Her body became and remained the means through which she expressed her emotional life—and her very identity—even after she married and had children. As she passed through the stages of adulthood, she began feeling that her naturally aging and imperfect body was no longer adequate. Meanwhile, all of her emotional stress continued to settle in and on her body. Purging seemed like the solution to maintain her looks, relieve her emotional tension and self-soothe. Soon she had full-blown bulimia and needed multiple rounds of treatment.

Louise says her recovery depended (and still depends) on finding ways to deal more directly with emotions, feel justified about having them, and express herself in constructive ways—instead of through her eating disorder. The result is a deeper intimacy in her relationships with her husband, her sons and even her parents. After years of work, she gained new understanding about her family dynamics, which in turn facilitated further emotional growth and insight. "For example, I used to think only negative feelings were taboo in my family," Louise says. "But now I realize that I really didn't know how to express positive ones either. At least for me, my family's happy-and-nice routine was a façade that wasn't really happy *or* nice."

Whether or not our parents are alive, we can't change the past. Nevertheless, residual issues, needs and disappointments in our relationships with our parents live on even after we become adults. Our families have the overwhelming and endless job of teaching us many incredibly complicated things about ourselves and life. As Louise's story illustrates, the family's toughest task is teaching us to understand and manage our emotional experience. In the families of eating-disordered women, this process is often blunted as parents model how to suppress emotion rather than express it. When individual feelings are not easily tolerated, anger, grief, anxiety, sadness, loss and other emotions just go underground.

But they can't stay there; they need an outlet. In a culture that pressures women to eat and look a certain way, it is easy for those emotions to be expressed through, or become intertwined with, how we manage food or our bodies. That's why identifying family patterns and dynamics is so crucial for eating disorder recovery.

Hungry for the Perfect Dad

Young or old, my clients tend to say similar things about their relationships with their fathers and/or stepfathers.

- He was/is angry and irritable.
- He was/is self-absorbed and inattentive to others' feelings.
- He didn't/doesn't seem capable of praising or acknowledging my achievements.
- He can't understand my issues about food or weight.
- He hates fat people and continually comments about women's bodies.
- He can't stand it when I fail to meet his standards.

As one patient said, "I'm in my fifties and I shouldn't still need my father's approval." But the fact remains that many of us suffer from what I call Father Hunger, the natural, universal and intrinsic longing for a connection to Dad.[5] When that hunger is not satisfied, we struggle with self-worth and self-confidence, and have more difficulty in our relationships with men and with life partners.

Many of my father-hungry clients interact with men, including their spouses, in ways very similar to how they interacted (or still interact) with their own fathers: avoiding issues in anticipation of anger; not expecting much in order to avoid feeling disappointed; feeling misunderstood, trivialized and unsure; and fearing the man's disapproval. These are unhealthy patterns at any age.

We can mistakenly believe that perfecting our bodies can fix the problems we have with our fathers, our partners, or other influential men in our lives. But they can't; trying to use our bodies to feed our Father Hunger only fuels disordered eating and appearance obsessions, and leaves our true needs and hungers unmet.

Dad and Relationships with Important People in Your Current Life

Take a few minutes to review the list of personal characteristics in the chart below. Mark the ones that applied (or apply) to your father or stepfather, and those that apply to your spouse, partner, or significant other. (You can also substitute a male authority figure, boss, colleague, friend, or any man with whom you have felt some difficulty.)

He is/was:	Dad/Stepdad	Partner
Often angry and irritable.		
Often self-absorbed and inattentive to others.		
Seldom able to praise or acknowledge your achievements.		
Seldom able to understand your issues about food or weight.		
Makes negative comments about women's bodies or about fat people.		
Often intolerant or impatient when others fail to meet his standards.		
Often avoids emotional issues or acts in ways to avoid his anger.		
I feel/felt:	Dad/Stepdad	Partner
Like I can seldom expect much from him.		
Unsure of myself around him.		
Misunderstood or trivialized by him.		
Like I regularly fear his disapproval.		
That my appearance, weight, or eating can please him.		

Compare how many characteristics apply to both your father and the important men in your current life. Now take a few minutes to write down your answers to the following questions.

- As a child, how did you feel about the problematic characteristics your father had?
- How do you feel about them now?
- What was your reaction to those characteristics as a girl?
- What is your reaction to them today?
- How closely (if at all) do your reactions to your father parallel the reactions you have to your spouse, partner, or other important men in your current life?

Write down your insights and share them in therapy or with a trusted friend to understand how you can begin to give up negative patterns and reinforce positive ones.

Hungry for the Perfect Mom

Even the best mother–daughter relationships are complicated. Sometimes we feel that Mom is smothering—too present in too many ways and making it difficult to differentiate ourselves as individuals. Some of us saw our Mom's passivity with Dad create an unhealthy family environment and a negative role model for us as growing girls. We hungered for examples of self-assertion, self-confidence and comfort with womanly appetites.

For some of us, the relationship with Mom was (or still is) dominated by concerns, competition and shared experiences around appearance, weight, dieting, shopping and "perfecting" one's body. These can never satisfy the deep hunger daughters and mothers have for intimacy. Instead, they feed a shallow and ultimately dangerous fixation on reshaping our bodies together rather than striving to connect our spirits.

Recovery and a healthy adulthood require that we set limits on Mom's influence, while claiming healthy autonomy and interdependence in our lives. Health and recovery also demand that we identify and legitimize our desires—including for food.

Observing our mothers' eating habits can help us to make sense of our own. Many of my patients manage to eat something for breakfast and dinner but never have lunch. They seem to be unable to tune into their bodies during the day. Often, as we discuss their relationship with food, they realize that they never saw their mothers eat lunch. Their mothers' inability to nourish themselves created an unconscious pattern for their own relationship with food as they aged.

Denying their midday hunger while quietly battling their bodies, mothers exacerbate their daughters' struggles to meet basic needs. If important women in our lives seem to deny their physical and spiritual hungers, it is difficult to imagine eating freely and enjoying our beautifully imperfect bodies in adulthood.

Patients from abusive or conflict-ridden homes often tell me that the only freely given nurturance came in the form of food. While everything else felt threatening or chaotic, Mom or Grandma cooked and served wonderful meals. Food was a refuge and the only positive expression of love. Years later, these women maintain a love-hate relationship with food, often punishing themselves by eating too much or too little.

Tracing the roots of our relationship with food and our body image can help us to be kinder and more forgiving to ourselves. The less self-blame we use, the easier it is to change our behaviors and develop better coping mechanisms.

Mom's Hand-Me-Downs

Many of our mothers channeled their frustrations and emotions into struggles with their bodies and food, creating a template for us as well. Take a look at the list below. Mark the characteristics that were (or are) true for your mother, and for you.

She often did or does:	Mom/ Stepmom	Me
Talk about her weight.		
Go on and off diets.		
Weigh herself.		
Complain about the changes in her weight or appearance as she aged.		
Enforce strict rules on eating.		
Keep many nonfat, low-fat, or other diet products in the house.		
Label foods as good or bad.		
Have secret stashes of candy or other special foods.		
Seem conflicted or in denial about her appetites and hungers.		
Express remorse or guilt after eating.		
Overeat or under-eat when she appeared upset.		
Appear unhappy or dissatisfied with herself.		
Encourage others to diet.		
Criticize my body.		
Maintain a standard of perfection for herself.		
Maintain a standard of perfection for me.		
Judge others based on their weight or appearance.		

If our moms spoke the language of fat, we are likely to speak it to ourselves and to our own children. Now run through the list again, and see what example you may be setting for your daughters, sons, or other young people in your life.

Whether we are young or old, we all want the same things from our mothers and our fathers—that is, to:

- feel wanted and accepted unconditionally
- feel respected as separate people
- be able to differ from them without losing them
- be acknowledged for who we are, not just for what we achieve
- feel good enough as is
- love and be loved.

We also crave these same feelings in our most important current relationships. Until we begin understanding and making peace with such powerful influences, we can't learn from them—and we may remain at their mercy. Fortunately, we *can* make peace with our past (and our parents), find harmony in ourselves, and nurture strong current and future relationships by taking time to recognize how our pasts are shaping our current lives.

The Shape of Our Current Family

The family we live in now also has a major effect on our body image, eating behavior and sense of self. The personalities of our partners and children weave together with our own continually developing identity and the old dynamics from our families of origin to create new family dynamics. These multiple and complex forces affect whether we have an eating or body image problem, whether our loved ones recognize the problem, whether they contribute to it (knowingly or not), and whether they can help us to recover from the problem.

Imposter Syndrome

In childhood, Meghan's family atmosphere was full of tension, unspoken emotions and endless demands. Most of the time, her father's authoritarian style, her mother's passivity and the family's high expectations for Meghan played out over meals, so food became symbolic and problematic for her.

As she grew up, Meghan developed impossibly high standards for herself so she never felt "good enough." Instead, she felt like an imposter frantically scrambling to keep from being discovered as a fraud. This degree of overdrive ultimately placed unbearable stress on Meghan's health, well-being and closest relationships.

Constantly pushing ourselves to do everything perfectly for everyone always backfires. We then can never truly meet anyone's needs, including our own. Nevertheless, many of us feel compelled to try and meet the impossible (therefore, unrealistic) standards we have set.

No matter how accomplished we actually are, we may feel like imposters. Because we are not perfect, we know that we are not what others think we are—or what we hope they think we are. Therefore, we simply do not believe, accept, or allow words and gestures of praise and affection. We maintain a distance that limits satisfaction and intimacy—for ourselves and others.

This merry-go-round is not merry at all, and it takes guts to decide to get off. Because we believe people value us only for what we do and how we look (not who we are), we also believe that accepting our imperfections will mean losing the affection or respect of others. But we are called "human beings" not human "doings" for a reason.[6] It is who we are inside that counts, not what we do or how we look outside. Isn't that what we tell our children?

In fact, our children actually benefit from imperfect parents. Girls in particular don't need mothers who set impossible standards for themselves. Children learn from what we do more than from what we say, and girls are particularly good observers of their moms and other important female role models. No matter what we tell them about being "good enough the way you are" and loving themselves, our words are meaningless if we cannot embrace our own imperfect humanity.

To be positive role models for our daughters and other young women, we have to relinquish the pursuit of perfection and live as genuine and honest beings. If we do this, we also will be liberated from living in fear of being "found out." Our loved ones will truly know us, and they'll actually love us *more* because they are getting the real thing, not some imposter.

If we never feel good enough or satisfied with ourselves, we cannot be open and available in our closest and most important relationships. Husbands and partners who want a trophy wife (rather than a real woman partner) don't deserve real women—and we don't deserve to have their warped standards influence how we value ourselves. A relationship based on trying to be someone we are not is no relationship at all. Real men and real women want to be with real women. As scary as it may be, when we let down our guard and risk being who we are inside, we offer our best to our intimate partners.

Perfectly Help-Less

Women are good at multitasking, but today's expectation that we can have it all by doing it all is simply a hoax. We cannot do all and be all without making ourselves vulnerable to stress-related illnesses and addictions. Something has to give; too often, it is us or our families.

We often believe that the perfect home, the perfect meals and the perfect body will create a perfect family. Trying to cross the ever shifting goal line of being good enough is impossible as we try to outdo our neighbors in living, looking and eating the "right" way.

Perfection is a myth; it simply doesn't exist (at least not in this world). Our appearance-first, perfectionist cultural and personal standards for women can sentence us to a life of despair and disconnection. When we strive to create that perfect family, real relationships suffer. Our spouses and children come to think that they are less important to us than symbols of perfection are. Like characters in "The Emperor's New Clothes," we pretend not to see the naked absurdity of trying to be Superwoman. Instead, our own lives become barren and naked as we obsess about being the ultimate wife, perfect mother, master employee and CEO chef.

I think perfectionism is based on the obsessive belief that if you run carefully enough, hitting each stepping-stone just right, you won't have to die. The truth is that you will die anyway and that a lot of people who aren't even looking at their feet are going to do a whole lot better than you, and have a lot more fun while they're doing it.[7]

Anne Lamott

Joan (whose story started this chapter) described a mother who gave but never expected to receive. She never learned to recognize, let alone meet, her own needs. How could she teach her children, especially her daughter, to identify, understand and satisfy their own hungers? In a healthy family, everyone, even a mother, is allowed to have needs, desires and hungers, and can expect to have at least some of them fulfilled.

Many of us have so many things going on in our lives, and so many areas where we are trying to prove ourselves. We believe we cannot take any time for ourselves—whether for the simplest of daily mental health breaks or for life-or-death recovery from an eating disorder. Yet when someone we love has a serious illness, or even a cold, we make time and support for them. We don't expect them to take care of themselves without any outside assistance—in fact, we insist on doing everything we can to help the healing process. We simply cannot be healthy if we continue to live by this double standard. We must practice what we preach when it comes to caring for ourselves and reaching out for the help we need.

Spouses and Partners

When it comes to our issues with weight, food and body image, most of us discover that spouses, partners and significant others can be part of the problem, part of the solution, or both. This is true whether our partners or spouses are male or female. Being the intimate partner of someone with an eating disorders is difficult, as one husband describes:

She's had several back surgeries and one abdominal surgery and I could wrap my head around those challenges. It was something I could see, touch, feel and understand. And, the eating disorder, I didn't. It made no sense to me. I was very angry about everything with it, and didn't understand where it was coming from or the underlying cause or reason. I couldn't grasp that.[8]

In addition, many partners struggle with the recovery process, because it is not as linear, logical, or predictable as recovery from back surgery. Male and female loved ones often ask me questions like "Can't you fix this eating disorder?" and "How long is this going to take?" I address their frustration directly by explaining how eating disorders are more complex than broken bones. I also stress that eating disorders are serious illnesses, not "simple" behaviors that can be speedily changed. I explain that both therapist and loved ones must adjust our expectations accordingly, understand recovery as a process and, whenever possible, work together as allies in healing.

Most adult women I work with have (or had) spouses or partners who fit into one of the following four types: the *Controller*, the *Codependent*, the *Clueless* and the *Committed*.

Controllers tends to be unrelenting in their demands on us. They may contribute to self-image problems by criticizing our bodies and dispensing approval only when we meet their standard for female beauty. They may criticize other areas of our lives, always wanting more and being dissatisfied with what we accomplish. Faced with these criticisms, we may use our bodies or eating to soothe ourselves or to feel a sense of personal control. Or we may believe that a perfect physique, diet, or style will finally please our partner.

Spouses and partners may also play the Controller during our recovery. They may want us to get better fast, and to do it their way, insisting on simplistic solutions like "Just eat!" Controllers may expect us to follow their recommendations for eating and exercise, asserting that they are the experts on our body. They may also try to control our treatment, imposing their beliefs, needs and timetable onto our therapeutic process. This approach interferes with our self-knowledge and is doomed to fail, but that may not stop a Controller.

Couples' therapy can often help with these hurdles. Some partners prefer to work through their issues in individual therapy or in a support group. The Controller needs to understand:

- what life experiences lead him or her to rely so heavily on control
- how his or her life is hampered by overreliance on control
- how to temper his or her over-controlling tendencies
- how his or her tendency to over control may exacerbate our eating and body image obsessions
- how his or her external control will hamper our ability to develop the *internal* control tools essential to recovery.

Raised to please others first, many women are tempted to just try to do what the Controller asks, but this will not work over the long run. Pretending to be better to please her partner is not the road to recovery, so it is critical to address these control issues.

The *Codependent* tends to be very needy and may come from an addictive family where children's needs weren't met. Codependent partners base their feelings, behaviors and view of reality on how another person behaves—or *might* behave. They sacrifice themselves to maintain the marriage or family equilibrium and avoid conflict. The Codependent may unknowingly contribute to our problems by discouraging changes that threaten the existing balance, even if those changes make us healthier, stronger or more independent—and stabilize the family. Uncertain how our recovery will change the rules of the relationship, Codependent partners may subtly resist even small changes, despite their genuine desire for us to get better. We may reinforce the Codependent response by avoiding conflict, blaming ourselves, and belittling our own needs.

When one partner has a serious problem like an eating disorder, it's very easy for the other partner to organize his or her life and self-worth around attempts to manage it, without realizing how this codependent reaction may help keep the problem going. A codependent couple builds their relationship on the problem (addiction, eating disorder and so forth), leaving little else to talk about or focus on. Marital, individual, or group therapy may help. If the Codependent is from an addictive family, Al-Anon[9] and/or Adult Children of Alcoholics/Dysfunctional Families[10] groups may also help.

Codependent's Checklist

Millions of people are affected by another person's eating or body image disorders. Read the statements listed in the chart below and check the ones that apply to your relationship with a sufferer.

I worry about someone else's eating behavior or appearance concerns.	
I tell lies to cover up for someone else's eating or appearance behaviors.	
If the person with eating or body image disorders really cared about me, she would stop her destructive behaviors.	
I blame her behavior on her relatives, friends, or companions.	
Plans, meals, or holidays are frequently upset, delayed, canceled, or spoiled because of her eating or body image problems.	
I make threats, such as, "If you don't start eating, I'll leave you."	
I secretly snoop around to discover whether she has been purging, restricting, or engaging in other dangerous eating behavior.	
I am afraid to upset her for fear it will set off an episode of purging, depression, or other problems.	
I've been hurt or embarrassed by her behavior.	
I search for hidden diet pills, laxatives and other tools of her disorder.	
I've refused social invitations out of fear or anxiety.	
I feel like a failure because I can't control her self-destructive behavior.	
I think that if she stopped her eating or body obsessions, our other problems would be solved.	
I have (even once) threatened to hurt myself to scare her.	
I feel angry, confused, or depressed most of the time.	
I feel there is no one who understands my problems or our situation.	

If you agreed with any of these statements, there is a very real possibility that you are responding in a codependent manner to your struggling loved one. Seek professional and other support in adopting the behaviors and attitudes most likely to support your loved one's recovery and your own well-being.

The *Clueless* spouse is often caring and loving, but simply hasn't taken the time or developed the skills to learn about women's experience today. Male partners are frequently stuck in a narrow worldview reinforced by the cultural straitjacket of masculinity. Often feeling inadequate and inept when it comes to understanding women, clueless spouses tend to avoid talking about or confronting personal or relationship problems.

They genuinely want us to be happy but aren't sure how to help, so they rarely inquire about our difficulties. Clueless partners tend to ignore and simplify issues, not knowing what questions to ask when they discover we are struggling. They may not be naturally inquisitive or intuitive either—remaining unaware that problems related to food or weight even trouble us, despite years of being together. They tend to be passive and to feel out of their comfort zone when dealing with sensitive, emotional issues. We may reinforce the Clueless response by covering up problems, hiding any sign of imperfection, and pretending that we are fine when we are not.

While both Joan's and Jennifer's spouses could be described as Clueless, they eventually did well in their efforts to support their wives' recovery after accepting a lot of direction from their wives and their therapists.

Like many women suffering from eating and body image issues, Joan and Jennifer were skeptical about involving their spouses in the recovery process. Both women's perfectionism made it hard for them to be seen as imperfect or needy. They also feared that their spouses might disappoint them by not caring or being unable to deliver. But their willingness to be open and honest paid off in the end.

Too often, we assume that our spouses or partners won't bother to understand or be able to help. However, most do care. They want to be involved but often don't know how to do it effectively. Once they understand the dimension of the problem and how they can help, Clueless, Co-Dependent or Controlling spouses blossom into Committed spouses, just as Joan's and Jennifer's did.

There is no problem that is not actually a gift.[11]

Elisabeth Kübler-Ross

The *Committed* spouse is able to support recovery, regardless of what it requires—and that requirement may be huge. Recovery sometimes brings major disruptions to a couple's life, especially if treatment requires the woman to leave home. Jobs must be put on hold and family obligations and child care rearranged, just as they would be for other serious or chronic illnesses. Committed spouses pitch in, shuffle their other commitments to share this burden, understand the depth of our problems, and recognize that there won't be any quick fix.

Louise's husband was surprised at how many people praised his commitment to his wife's treatment, which included residential treatment in a facility hundreds of miles away from their home. He said:

> I love her and was ready to do anything to save her. In my mind, I had no choice. This is exactly what I would have done had she been physically ill with cancer. All of us, Louise, me, the kids, did what we had to do. Sometimes, there wasn't a lot of support for the level of commitment we made, because there is still a lot of stigma surrounding emotional and psychiatric problem, especially eating disorders. Plus, contemporary culture promotes the idea that we should throw away a relationship as soon as it isn't perfect anymore, or we run into troubles. I'm glad we did it the way we did, and that we all have Louise back.[12]

After being sick for more than half of her life, Louise wonders if she would have recovered without her spouse's devotion, acceptance, and his openness to changing his life so she could concentrate on her treatment.

Any spouse can move from being Controller, Codependent or Clueless to being a Committed partner. It requires being open and willing to admit imperfections and beginning to deal with difficult emotions. Some women fear that their spouses or partners will disappoint or reject them, so they deny their loved ones the opportunity to truly know them and what they need. Ironically, we give a precious gift to our partners when we ask for their help. Our partners and friends need our help in order to help us.

The fear that our relationship will change if we get better can keep us stuck for a long time. We question if we'll be discarded once we reveal our true selves. Our spouses or partners may wonder if they will still be needed, once we get well. It is important to remember that all relationships change (because all relationships are at least a little fluid) whether we get better or not, but remaining stuck in our old ways creates increasing distance between us. This distance may look very comfortable and familiar, but if we are changing anyway, why not work to bring more honesty, spontaneity and health into our lives and relationships?

Intimacy

Eating and body disorders inevitably destroy our most intimate relationships, both physically and psychologically. For instance, when we don't eat enough, the body's evolutionary hardwiring triggers a plunge in our libido—because sexual activity can lead to pregnancy, which in turn consumes energy that may be scarce during famine. As you saw in Chapter 2, the body interprets food restriction as a sign of famine and quickly adapts to protect itself. (The flip side? Eating a balanced diet and getting sufficient calories is often the best tonic for low libido—a natural Viagra for modern women.) It takes time, but many women get past the uncomfortable feelings of fullness during the recovery process.

Instead of sharing a relaxing meal at home or in a restaurant, eating with our partner becomes measured (literally and figuratively) and devoid of pleasure. Any break in routine, even an evening out or weekend away, becomes a major stressor. For some couples, depression and hopelessness set in as their world shrinks to fit inside the narrow limits of restricted eating and joyless body obsessions. Life is no longer fun the way we or our partner once imagined.

In addition to sapping sexual energy, despair and depression about body image also psychologically disconnect us from opportunities to enjoy physical contact. If we cannot tolerate our bodies, we cannot enjoy anyone else touching them or seeking closeness with them. We may allow some sexual contact because we are afraid of being rejected or of disappointing our partners. But this contact is more likely to bring us conflict than satisfaction, joy or pleasure. Our partners often sense this, even if we don't.

Eating disorders therapist Nancy Albus tells the story of a new client who reported that her sex life was normal. A week later, while talking with the woman's husband, Albus asked for his perspective. "Well," he replied sadly, "if you think making love with the shades pulled, the lights out and her clothes on is normal, then yes, I suppose our sex life is normal."[13]

Keenly aware of our body's imperfections, we feel negative, worthless, devoid of sexuality, or ashamed of any sexual appetite. Shame over past abuse or violation can add to any anxiety or fear we feel in our present relationships, no matter how safe and loving our current partner is.

Creating an atmosphere of openness and honesty is the best way to improve intimacy. This takes time, trust, support, practice and sometimes professional guidance. The strength of couples who love each other unconditionally, and commit themselves to working through such daunting obstacles is awesome and inspiring.

When Tracy first came to me for psychotherapy, she didn't meet the medical criteria for anorexia or bulimia. But she still spent years battling multiple conflicts with food, weight, body image and exercise. Tracy was 35, recently remarried, and couldn't figure out why her problem was getting worse. Tracy felt her first marriage in her 20s failed because both she and her ex were too young, immature and inexperienced. She coped well with her divorce, pursued a career and graduate school, and was now with a new husband. She loved Tom deeply and saw him as her soul mate.

Despite this, Tracy started to feel more depressed in the months after her wedding. To make herself feel better, she exercised more, ate more rigidly, and obsessed about every aspect of her appearance. She even took laxatives and vomited every now and then when she felt desperate and fat.

Used to handling things on her own, Tracy was not instantly comfortable in therapy. But gradually she revealed a history of childhood sexual abuse by a close family friend. She had never talked about this before; even her parents and sisters did not know. After each incident, and whenever she was upset about the abuse, Tracy used strenuous physical activity—usually running or biking—as her way to cope with her overwhelming emotions and anxiety. As she proceeded through high school and college, she obsessed about her weight and appearance, sometimes restricting, bingeing, or vomiting when these feelings swelled up.

While this behavior was disruptive to her, no one else expressed concern. Indeed, other people complimented her appearance and her strict exercise schedule. Only recently had Tom questioned the frequency of her exercise and the rigidity of her eating habits. Despite this new and loving marriage to her soul mate, Tracy's symptoms felt more out of control than ever before.

As her relationship with Tom deepened, Tracy felt increasing shame about her past and tremendous anxiety about the possibility that her future children might be abused themselves. Tracy gradually explored her sexual abuse history and uncovered her fear that any intimate partner who discovered her past would reject her as damaged goods. Despite their deep trust in each other, Tracy feared that even Tom might react this way. Consequently, the marriage's growing intimacy paradoxically fueled Tracy's anxiety and self-loathing—causing her body obsessions to multiply.

Eventually, Tracy agreed to have Tom join in therapy sessions, where she bravely risked telling him about her abuse. Tom's emotions ran the gamut from sadness to rage at how badly Tracy had been hurt. He was especially angry that her family never recognized or prevented it. Despite these powerful impulses, Tom assured Tracy that he could handle his feelings, would do anything he could to help her and would not leave her. Tom even understood when Tracy said she needed to back off from their sexual relationship temporarily while she worked through her feelings about the abuse.

Tom worked hard to understand how childhood sexual abuse damages adults and their partners. He read books and got information from self-help organizations and the Internet.[14] He accepted my recommendation that he see a therapist to help him with his anger at Tracy's perpetrator and her family. Worried that they would be too upset by it, Tracy did not want to share the abuse with her parents. However, she did talk to her sisters, who responded with tremendous support and validation. Tracy feels closer to them and to Tom than she ever has. She also has forgiven her parents for not realizing what went on all those years ago.

Tracy has been able to heal in large part because Tom stood by her and remained committed to her and to their marriage. They now have a family of their own, and she is managing her anxiety about protecting her children. She no longer does anything harmful to her body, although appearance and exercise are still very important to her.

Tracy's story shows a universal truth: when it comes to body image and relationships with food, the family is an asset, a liability, or (usually) both. Whether we examine our family of origin, current family or extended family, we find forces that can help or hinder us in the search for a peaceful relationship with body, weight and food.

Surviving Eating Disorders and Body Image Despair: Ten Steps for Spouses, Partners and Other Loved Ones

1. **Eating disorders and body image obsessions have tremendous power over your loved one.** She isn't trying to hurt you and she isn't being resistant or stubborn out of spite. These are her own survival techniques and at times they will overpower her logic and will. Recognize the disease's power and don't take her obsessions personally.

2. **Be compassionate.** She feels deep pain that she can only articulate through her body. Hopefully, in time she will have words for her emotions.

3. **Your loved one and her illness are not the same thing.** Remember and repond to the person who is covered up by these obsessions—she is still the person you love. Help her to recognize herself as well.

4. **Help her to see that there is more to her, you and life than food, weight and appearance.** Talk about other issues. Don't let the eating and body obsessions dominate your interactions and conversations.

5. **Admit your own anger, frustration and helplessness.** Talk to others in similar circumstances. Join a support group for family members or spouses of people suffering from body image and eating problems. Read supportive books and visit support groups online for help and encouragement.

6. **Consider getting help for yourself.** You will feel overwhelmed, discouraged, tired and angry at times. Working with a professional can help you to manage these feelings and deal with them constructively.[15]

7. **You are her partner, not her treatment team.** No matter how much you love her, you cannot turn her problems around alone. Resist the impulse to battle over weight, food and exercise. Help her to find a therapist, dietitian, physician and/ or treatment program so she has professional help guiding her.

8. **Ask how you can help, and listen for the answer. At times, you can only be in the background, conveying love and support.**

Other times, she may need more direct help from you. This may be confusing, but she needs to be in charge of how you help her.

9. **These problems don't disappear overnight, no matter how hard someone works in therapy or how good a treatment program is.** Recovery is a long, winding road with lots of bumps and potholes. Don't expect her to be perfect in her recovery. Help her to take one day at a time—you do the same!

10. **Logic doesn't work: love does.** Endless debates about food, health, exercise, or weight do more harm than good. Helping her to feel that she is loved and that life is worth living will do more than a thousand reasoned arguments. Some women who have recovered believe that the love and hope of their significant other is what made them hope and believe that they could survive without the life preserver of their eating disorders and body obsessions.

Notes

1 *A Woman's Conflict: The Special Relationship Between Women and Food* (Englewood, NJ: Prentice-Hall, 1980) p. 10.
2 "Protecting children from self-loathing thoughts." Media Planet. See www.modernwellnessguide.com/lifestyle/protecting-children-from-self-loathing-thoughts (retrieved September 25, 2015).
3 Joe Kelly, *Dads & Daughters: How to Inspire, Support and Understand Your Daughter* (New York: Broadway, 2003) p. 112.
4 *You Can Observe a Lot by Watching: What I've Learned about Teamwork from the Yankees and Life* (Hoboken, NJ: Wiley, 2009).
5 Margo Maine, *Father Hunger: Fathers, Daughters, and the Pursuit of Thinness* (Second Edition) (Carlsbad, CA: Gürze Books, 2004).
6 I first heard this phrase from my dear friend Reverend Dr. Steve Emmett, who points this out frequently.
7 *Bird by Bird: Some Instructions on Writing and Life* (New York: Anchor, 1995) p. 28.
8 Interview with Joe Kelly, 2014.
9 See www.al-anon.org.
10 See www.adultchildren.org.
11 *The Wheel of Life: A Memoir of Living and Dying* (New York: Scribner, 1998) p. 233.
12 Personal correspondence with Margo Maine, 2014.
13 Personal conversation with Joe Kelly, 2014.
14 For more, see Laura Davis, *Allies in Healing: When the Person You Love Was Sexually Abused as a Child* (New York: William Morrow, 1991).
15 Visit http://www.joekelly.org/coaching-for-men, where my co-author Joe Kelly provides online coaching for loved ones. This coaching provides information about eating disorders, and how loved ones can best support treatment and recovery—while also handling their own frustration with the disorder's process.

7 The New Extended Family

How Culture Shapes Us

The female body is the place where this society writes its messages.[1]
Rosalind Coward

Women's widespread discontent with their body image is a sociocultural phenomenon that varies profoundly from culture to culture. For example, rotund women are considered more desirable as wives in some parts of the world, so women strive to be big and some families strive to make girls fat. A 2013 research study found that almost a quarter of women in Mauritania reported being force fed as a child. Meanwhile, 32 percent of women and 29 percent of men in this impoverished Saharan country approved of the practice.[2]

Force-feeding looks like an eerie mirror image of anorexia. Why do women do it? Apparently for the same reason Western women do. As Jidat Mint Ethmane of Mauritania told the *Wall Street Journal*, "Beauty is more important than health."[3]

The point is that our pursuit of a perfect shape is neither timeless nor inevitable. Instead, it is driven by external (and frequently arbitrary) cultural standards. So why does it feel like a universal truth?

A major factor is the way that culture (especially in the form of the media and marketing) has taken over many functions that the extended family provided for earlier generations of women. In the past, relatives had a profound influence on a woman's nuclear family and her individual identity. For millennia, grandparents, cousins, aunts, uncles, neighbors and friends helped raise children, passing along ancestral expectations and values.

That was often a good thing, sometimes a bad thing and usually a mixture of positive and negative.

When our great-grandmothers were girls, they usually spent little time away from their own grandmothers and great aunts—an arrangement that might have felt downright stifling some days. But, our 19th-century female ancestors probably also demonstrated (in word and deed) what the family valued most in women and girls: integrity, hard work, caring for others and commitment to family. Rigid external standards of beauty seldom made the list because (in the days before the onset of mass electronic media) they were seldom relevant to survival or satisfaction.

The Culture as Extended Family

> The more we come to depend on the images offered to us by those who try to distract us, entertain us, use us for their own purposes, and make us conform to the demands of a consumer society, the easier it is for us to lose our identity. These imposed images actually make us into the world they represent.[4]
>
> Father Henri Nouwen, Ph.D.

Western culture remains ambivalent about the potential, power and changing role of contemporary women. Our increasing influence is met by an ongoing backlash of shifting and unattainable standards of beauty and behavior that keep most women on edge and anxious about how others see us. In an earlier book, I coined the term Body Wars[5] to define this systematic and relentless assault on our bodies by the economic and social systems that benefit from suppressing women's economic and social power.

Because these assaults are so normal in our culture, we are unsure of ourselves and of what we really hunger or yearn for, no matter what our age. Instead of celebrating and pursuing our appetites, many of us joylessly pursue the perfect body. Meanwhile, our culture celebrates our pursuit of perfection because it erodes our capacity to realize the broader influence and power we can attain.

A hundred years ago, it was hard (although still possible) for a woman to escape her extended family and its standards, even though she could never entirely escape its influence on her development. In today's very mobile society, the influence of *human* extended family is fading. Many of us no longer live near our families of origin. Even if we remain geographically close, we are likely to be wrapped up in the modern woman's life of multiple and demanding roles, leaving little time to spend with relatives. We may not even realize the degree to which we miss the soothing, ageless wisdom that springs from deep family connections and the informal mentoring provided by older women in our communities.

Of course, the nuclear family still plays a major role in creating our identity and guiding our development, but today's media-saturated culture has usurped much of the influence once held by extended families. Indeed, the culture may sometimes be even more powerful than the nuclear family in a woman's life.

Few Western women can escape 21st-century media and marketing's promotion of myths about the body and perfection. Every day, this culture-as-extended-family tells us that the most important and valuable thing about a woman is her external appearance. That's a radically different message from the one our ancestors got from their extended families at the turn of the 20th century.

For instance, none of our foremothers had to master nonstop media. This is another example of the way that we are immigrants into a foreign way of living life as women. Corporate-owned media culture is more inescapably *with* us than the human extended family was with our grandparents.

- As soon as we wake, we check our phones or tablets and turn on radios or TVs. Our very first morning movement may be turning off the alarm on our smart phone. Before we know it, we are online.
- We wear clothing with prominent logos and other marketing messages.
- Data from billboards, phone screens and earbuds crowd our ride to and from work.
- Unbidden ads pop up on our tablets and computers.
- Ads literally envelop the food we eat for lunch.
- Back home at night, we scan mobile devices and flip through countless videos and TV shows until we drop off to sleep.

Coursing through nearly every vessel of this commercial media octopus is the message that we don't measure up to the modern ideal of perfect beauty. The culture's values and expectations about us as women are authoritarian, rigid and unreasonable—just the way authoritarian parents and grandparents can be. But while you can negotiate with your parents (and even your extended family), you can't negotiate with the inanimate screens and other "smart" technologies.

More often than we realize, smart technology delivers hyperactive, loud, overbearing, manipulative and nonstop marketing and other messages from the culture, telling us who to be and what to do, regardless of who it is we actually are or what it is we actually need. On the occasions that we recognize the absurdity of these notions, we might feel tempted to shout back at our screens in frustration. But Siri won't really listen. We never get a chance to say anything personal to our electronic companions, or to hear them respond to who we truly are.

Facing such an unrelenting and rigid assault on our self-worth, even the hardiest among us sometimes succumb to self-doubt and self-hatred. No matter how absurd it is to expect a 65-year-old woman to look like a 15-year-old girl, women of every age feel their value measured by a commercially generated standard of beauty.

The more eagerly we pursue perfection, the more we feel the need to buy products and services that we don't really need. There is enormous profit in making us feel bad about ourselves—but no *financial* gain in appreciating ourselves, our loved ones and our shared imperfections. In the cultural extended family, creating profit is exponentially more important than nurturing the human extended family. Unique family stories that help us cherish our heritage create no financial revenue, but bring huge profits in dignity and self-worth.

So while familial ties of the human extended family (as well as religion and community) are weakening, we must fight internal battles over body image, because the media, culture and consumer value system are relentlessly assailing our bodies, well-being and self-respect.

Bodies of the Nineteenth and Twentieth Centuries

> Renoir once said that were it not for the female body, he never could have become a painter. This is clear: there is love for women in each detail of the canvas, and love for self, and there is joy, and there is a degree of sensual integration that makes you want to weep, so beautiful it seems, and so elusive.[6]
>
> Caroline Knapp

While today's framework of beauty may seem cast in stone, a look back across modern history shows that it isn't. Find a photograph or a print of a Pierre-Auguste Renoir painting in an encyclopedia, art history book or online. You'll quickly see how differently we experience the female shape today than women and men did little more than a century ago, when Renoir was in his prime. For example, his 1910 *After the Bath*[7] shows how Renoir celebrated the sensuality and sexual attraction of a large, fertile woman. This was the cultural ideal beauty when our great- and great-great-grandmothers were in their prime.

However, these same ancestors might never have seen an original Renoir woman or even a print of one, because they lived in the last decades before electronic mass media exploded into our culture. Without radio, TV, or the Internet, they had radically different interactions with the culture, themselves and the very concept of body image. Our great-grandmothers:

- were never exposed to thousands of mass media images every day
- often lived without mirrors
- lived in an economy that did not depend on them spending money daily to alleviate their body discontent
- saw relatives, friends, neighbors and other real women with diverse body shapes far more frequently than they saw idealized advertising images.

As a result, it was less common for turn-of-the-century women to be concerned if their bodies did not measure up to Renoir's plump models.[8] The very notion of American women comparing themselves to mass-marketed beauty standards was as foreign as Renoir's France. Our great-grandmothers spent vastly more of their time looking at real people in their natural extended families and neighborhoods than they ever did looking at ads, newspapers, magazines and other commercially produced imagery. Their community culture held much less rhyme or reason for obsessing about body shape.

When the first fashion shows and beauty pageants began in the early 20th century, participants averaged 50 pounds more than they do today—and were still considered the height of beauty. The ensuing decades mark an epoch of increasing attacks on women's bodies though pervasive media marketing which touts the latest product or procedure to "perfect" our bodies—and promotes the notion that our ultimate value is our appearance.

The year 1920 was a pivotal one in media history and women's history. The first radio broadcast reported the presidential election results, and within a decade, millions of homes had radio sets. Coming less than three months after ratification of the Nineteenth Amendment, the 1920 election was also the first to include women voters nationwide. But almost immediately, this growth in women's rights was met with a cultural backlash. During the Roaring Twenties, the Miss America pageant began and popular beauty standards shifted to the thinner flapper image, with bound breasts and a penchant for "slimming" (what we call dieting).

While women's movements continued to challenge traditions throughout the 20th century, archaic narrow standards for female beauty remained entrenched. For example, with the help of rapidly expanding mass media, fashion took on a more central role in women's lives.

When so-called second wave feminism generated major social change in the 1960s and 1970s, the beauty ideal shrunk from buxom, full-hipped Marilyn Monroe to matchstick Twiggy (5' 6" and 90 pounds—about 70 percent of the expected weight for her height and age). Fashion spreads and magazine covers favored models with the "starved" look. Weight Watchers and the dieting craze took off, joining the fashion industry to foster women's uncertainty about our worth. By the millions, we started looking for answers to life's questions in the mirror, on the scale and amid the clothing racks.

By the late 1970s, US women had won legal access to education, birth control and sexual freedom unimagined by earlier generations of women. But while the opportunities to fulfill these appetites widened, our basic body appetites often remained taboo. Social liberation brought intense body shame and sanctions.

For example, only a tiny fraction of today's Miss America contestants fall in a healthy ratio of weight-to-height. In fact, 60 percent of these young women fit a long-held parameter for anorexia: less than 85 percent of the expected weight for their height.[9] Pageant contestants average 14 hours of exercise per week, with some working out as many as 35 hours.[10] Their bodies are unnaturally crafted, sculpted and starved in a subculture where fasting and purging are normal.

Today, the average US woman is 5' 4" tall and weighs 164 pounds. The average fashion model is 5' 10" and 107 pounds, with a BMI of 15.4.[11] We can trace some of that change to a slightly higher average weight for women, but most of the difference lies in a shrinking of the standard model of perfection—who is hardly a prototype for women likely to throw their weight around in order to exercise power. The gap between real and ideal continues to widen, festering great discontent for many women.

A few brave models with fuller (in reality, more normal bodies), like Emme, Kate Dillon, Amy Lemons, Crystal Renn and Carrie Otis show the guts to question the tyrannical standards of beauty, raise public consciousness about body image and eating disorders, and still succeed in their chosen profession. They courageously share stories of how they were pressured and threatened to shape their bodies into something smaller than their natures intended. These pioneers are admirable, but the fashion industry isolates them as so-called plus-sized models, even though their weight-height proportions are just plain average.

When the high profile Ford modeling agency closed its "plus size" division in 2013, Gary Dakin and Jaclyn Sarka lost their jobs. So, they founded the Jag model agency and took the revolutionary step of representing women regardless of their size. Discarding the traditional path of relegating "plus size" models to a separate sub-industry, Jag incorporates them across the spectrum, placing models of all sizes in ads and on the cover of magazines.[12]

Meanwhile, France, Israel, Italy and Spain have taken an even more revolutionary step by legally banning the use of emaciated models. Many activists and organizations, like the National Eating Disorders Association and the Academy for Eating Disorders, have advocated for similar legislation in the US, However, the Council of Fashion Designers of America consistently opposes the idea, saying that the eating disorders awareness and health guidelines it sends to members of the industry each season are sufficient.[13]

Today, only a rebellious woman is likely to feel positive when her mirror reveals Renoir's ideal of ample, fertile, feminine contours. Instead, we are encouraged to feel ashamed if we look older, softer, rounder, or curvaceous. The body type dictated by our genes and ethnic roots has no relevance and gets no respect. By today's "Perfect Body" standards, beauty is:

- singular, not diverse
- thin, not full
- crafted, not natural
- bought, not innate
- hard, bony and muscular—like a boy with breasts.

Women are expected (and we expect ourselves) to judge our worth by arbitrary external beauty standards, while also assuming new social roles and work responsibilities. We want to feel part of the extended family that the culture represents. We want its approval as well. No wonder we feel tired, confused and distressed, ever willing to manipulate our bodies endlessly, in hopes of feeling good enough.

> This cause is not altogether and exclusively women's cause. It is the cause of human brotherhood as well as human sisterhood, and both must rise and fall together. Women cannot be elevated without elevating man, and man cannot be depressed without depressing women also.[14]
>
> Frederick Douglass

Women and Wanting

A booming consumer culture requires that women want to buy; in fact, we make 85 percent of all purchases in the United States.[15] Since our economy thrives on our purchases, it depends on manufacturing female desire—even if that manufactured desire puts us at war with our own bodies.

Consumer culture exploded in the 1950s after World War II, when factories switched from war materials to consumer products. Many women lost their manufacturing jobs to returning soldiers; they were sent home to manufacture desire for the flood of new consumer goods. The number of magazines, broadcasters and other advertising channels grew exponentially, pressuring women to want the perfect home and all the products needed to complete a "perfect" family picture.

By the late 1990s, shopping malls made up over four billion square feet in the United States—about 16 square feet per person. By 2010, two-thirds of US mall shoppers were women; and about 48 percent of mall sales take place in apparel stores[16] (demonstrating how heavily malls rely on women's drive to be fashionable). In order to support all of this shopping space, retailers need each of us to want a lot so that we'll purchase a lot. From many directions, we feel compelled to buy.

For example, within days of the September 11, 2001 terrorist attacks, our leaders said that the most patriotic thing to do was shop. Enshrined as a fundamental American identity and value, conspicuous consumption would stabilize our culture, prove our strength and keep the terrorists from defeating us. After decades of reinforcement, we've accepted that a central female role is to shop and consume. While this is very good for our market economy's profit makers, it doesn't work so well for women's self-worth or our access to economic or political power. The more time, money and energy we spend shopping, the less we invest in the activities that will bring us personal authority and gender equity.

The Power of Money

Over the past century, women have gained (through our own will and effort) unheralded advances in choice, opportunity, schooling, responsibility, money, expectations and influence. But we are still far from having equal status.

The consequences are not theoretical. Some are absurd—such as sales tax policies in 40 states which categorize tampon and menstrual pad sales as non-essential purchases.[17] Other inequalities are far more costly.

Women still earn about 23 percent less than men for comparable work (and have fewer benefits). We must work 60 extra days each year to make the same money a man makes.[18] Poverty rates among women in the US are substantially above the poverty rates for men. More than one in seven US women—nearly 18 million—lived in poverty in 2013. More than half of all poor children lived in families headed by women.[19]

Nevertheless, we spend a much higher percentage of our earnings on our appearance than men do. We invest in cosmetics, beauty rituals, dieting, clothing, surgery and other attempts to perfect our looks in the hopes of earning status, acceptance and self-worth. The market for so-called aesthetic procedures such as body contouring, skin tightening and cellulite reduction is anticipated to grow at double digit compound annual rates through 2018.[20] The more we submit to judging our worth by the world's standards about external appearance, the less power we have to make the world a better place for women—and for the men and children with whom we share this planet.

A Fashion is nothing more than an induced epidemic.[21]

George Bernard Shaw

Madison Avenue steers our purchases in trivial directions and relentlessly objectifies and pseudosexualizes the female body to sell goods and services. Marketers co-opt women's movement language to sell the idea that a *product* will liberate or strengthen us as women. We are supposed to get "New Freedom" from maxi pads, desirability from alcohol and rebellious power from tobacco.

The prevailing consumer culture leads us to believe that our power lies in purchasing. Now that we have our own money, we can join this new wave of consumer feminism and buy more of everything—bigger cars, houses and wardrobes—for us and for our families. But these narrow choices are empty of the real nourishment our lives and spirits need. Drowning in the sea of marketing, we lose any inkling of what we really thirst for. Do we want a pair of designer heels to make us look taller and thinner—or do we want time to reflect, the power to influence legislation, and a chance to hold hands with a child, friend, or lover? Do we seriously think that the sisterhood of sharing community power can really be replaced by the sisterhood of shopping?

Ad Addiction

Advertising and marketing are the engines of consumer culture. Many of us say (and believe): "Advertising doesn't influence *me*." Such assertions are naive at best and self-destructive at worst. Corporations would not stay in business long if they spent billions of dollars on marketing that didn't prompt us to buy. During 2016, marketers will spend more than $200 billion on advertising in the United States alone[22]—because it works. Marketing expert Jean Kilbourne, PhD, argues convincingly that the sophistication and ubiquity of today's advertising asserts an addictive power over people in a consumer culture.[23] Marketing's multimedia, subliminal and persistent methods get us to believe that a purchase can perfect our lives by providing meaning and fulfillment.

Remember that a century ago, many women only rarely saw an advertisement, as they lived their daily lives with little mass media (none of it electronic). Today we rarely experience a minute without marketing's intrusion into our psyche. The average Western woman is exposed to as many as 3,000 ads a day[24]—more than three a minute during normal waking hours. That volume of consumption is extreme and makes our new extended "family" look very much like an addicted family.

Your Personal Ad Volume

Here's a simple single-day exercise to create awareness of how deeply advertising enters our lives. When you wake up tomorrow, start keeping close track of the amount of time when there is no marketing or advertising within sight or within earshot. Be sure to count any time spent when brand names and logos are visible, and be sure to include scenarios like these.

- You are driving in the country, far away from billboards, out of cell phone range, and with the radio off—while the name and/ or logo of the car you are driving is still visible on the steering wheel or dashboard.
- You spend hours in the library, where publisher's logos are visible on the spines and covers of books.
- You wear pieces of clothing (including shirts, pants, shoes, jackets, and so forth) that feature highly visible logos and/or names of the clothing brand, a school, sports team, or other entity.

At the end of the day, add up the time you spent free from any form of marketing. We've done this experiment, and our free time amounted to less than an hour. The exercise is not designed as an indictment of marketing, but rather as a way to raise personal awareness of marketing's ubiquity in our lives.

Marketing imagery bombards us with increasing speed and intensity, making them nearly impossible to screen or filter before they are absorbed into our consciousness. As recently as 20 years ago, 30-second television commercials routinely had only a handful of edits; an image or shot could last 10, 15, or even the entire 30 seconds. Next time you watch TV, count the number of edits or shots in today's commercials. Most 30-second spots now have 40 or 50 different shots, with images lasting a split second while machine-gunned into our heads.[25] Meanwhile, TV commercials are now only a fraction of the average person's marketing diet. Pop-up and other ads crowd websites and smartphone apps. Marketers "embed" products and name brands into videogames, television programming and editorial content, blurring the line between ads and everything else.[26] We are left without enough time, context, or information to analyze, consider and decide whether to accept or reject this flood of marketing messages.

Most of us grew up watching television and were exposed to ads before we could even talk, but each year, marketing intrudes ever more deeply into our children's lives. While a small handful of advocacy groups like the Campaign for Commercial Free Childhood (www. commercialfreechildhood.org) try to stem that tide, we seldom speak up against the worsening waves of marketing directed at adult women. No one seems to care that women of all ages, shapes, colors and ethnicities are told to look like skinny, fair-skinned preteens. We spend years of our lives drenched in these "perfect" images—they seep into the pores of our consciousness, subliminally shaping our decisions and perceptions. They ruthlessly attack our connection to our bodies, desires and feelings—in the relentless pursuit of profit.

The formula for profit at women's magazines requires that the content of the magazine makes each reader feel like she doesn't measure up alongside articles and ads that promise she will fit in or feel better about herself if she buys an advertised product. The more the content drives *down* readers' self-esteem, the more it drives *up* magazine profits. The formula has worked for decades and is backed up by psychological research showing that the self-esteem of women and girls drops markedly after only a few minutes of reading a fashion magazine.[27]

Most of the female images in ads and on the screen are not even real; they are computer "enhanced" (more accurately, computer distorted). Many of these mythical images are composites, incorporating the features of several different people. We mistake these pretty images as our perfect ideal, when they are not even real women.

> If you retain nothing else, always remember the most important rule of beauty, which is: who cares?[28]
>
> Tina Fey

Big Questions

The next time you feel the desire to look like a media image of a "perfect" woman, ask yourself if she looks strong enough to do any of these.

- Work in the fields?
- Operate machinery?
- Carry a child?
- Nurse the sick?
- Defend herself against sexual assault?
- Change a tire?
- Play professional sports?
- Compete with men in the boardroom or factory floor?
- Coach a soccer team?
- Run for Congress—or maybe even President?

Next, ask yourself:

- Is it possible that smaller women are less of a threat to the status quo?
- Is it really possible to eat less but be more?

Even incredibly accomplished women are stuck in the pursuit of perfection, spending immense energy, anxiety and cash trying to change their bodies. For example, Madeleine K. Albright's vast achievements as the first female US Secretary of State were fueled by intense pride in her Slavic heritage. Yet, her autobiography describes how Albright felt chronically insecure inside the short, stocky shape of her Slavic body.[29] The memoir relates continual concerns about weight, but includes no acknowledgment of how absurd it is for the country's most powerful diplomat to agonize over her natural appearance.

Many of us feel the same way: proud of our family but ashamed of the body that very same family gave us. The desire to feel more accepted by our culture dominates our daily lives, and fuels an unconscious civil war between our body and our sense of self.

Lookism and Ageism

Our culture equates age with sickness, dependence and helplessness, apparently blind to the millions of people who actively enjoy dynamic aging. Hundreds of thousands of older people travel to hostels and RV campgrounds, join exercise programs, return to school, or start second careers. With the media focus on deterioration rather than vitality, we lose sight of these facts about older residents of the United States:

- Women reaching age 65 have an *average* life expectancy of 20 additional years.[30]
- Forty-seven percent of women aged 75 and older live on their own.[31]
- A mere two percent of people age 65 to 84 live in nursing homes.[32]
- Only 14 percent of Americans age *85 or older* live in nursing homes.[33]
- A full 80 percent of adults 45 and over say they want to remain in their current home and local community as they age.[34]

Almost 70 percent of voters over 65 (many of them mobilized by AARP, one of the nation's most powerful political forces) go to the polls, while only about a third of younger voters do.[35]

> Fair-skinned blacks invented "passing" as a term, Jews escaping anti-Semitism perfected the art, and the sexual closet continues the punishment, but pretending to be a younger age is probably the most encouraged form of "passing," with the least organized support for coming out as one's true generational self.[36]
>
> Gloria Steinem

While life expectancy increases, our ideas about aging and human potential remain stunted. As we move from our 20s into our 30s, 40s, 50s, 60s and beyond, we see fewer and fewer women like us in the media and popular culture.

Candace Bergen's 2015 memoir[37] drew wide attention for challenging this reality. The Emmy winner, Oscar® nominee and former supermodel confessed that, at age 68, she's happy being "fat" and loves to eat. If women over 50 typically have to choose between preserving either their face or their butts, she happily choses the former. Bergen writes: "At a recent dinner party I shared bread and olive oil, followed by chocolate ice cream with my husband. A woman near me looked at me, appalled, and I thought, 'I don't care.'" Watching her contemporaries struggle to remain thin reinforces Bergen's determination to do what is right for her.

Bergen's most famous role remains iconic because similar portrayals remain unusual. Murphy Brown was a newly sober, 40-something TV journalist and anchor who, Bergen writes, "cared not a whit what others thought of her. That character gave me permission to be my brattiest, bawdiest self."[38] The decade-long comedy premiered in 1988 after creator Diane English resisted CBS's demands to rewrite Brown for a younger actress. Four years later, the character became a single mother and unexpectedly took center stage in the 1992 US Presidential campaign, when Vice-President Dan Quayle criticized the fictional Brown for "ignoring the importance of fathers by birthing a child alone."[39] Bergen writes that "Diane had created a complex, original, endearing, feisty, take-no-prisoners woman," and gave Bergen her first experience of throwing herself into a role "with such abandon and joy." The Murphy Brown character was far from perfect, and in real life, Bergen is not surrendering to the pressure to be perfect.

The longest tenure of a *nonfictional* female anchor on prime time network is less than five years: Katie Couric on CBS (2006–2011) and Diane Sawyer on ABC (2009–2014). Both were replaced by men. Barbara Walters (1976–1978) and Elizabeth Vargas (six months in 2009) co-anchored with a man on ABC before the network reverted to the male-only format. The NBC Nightly News has never had a regular female anchor or co-anchor. Meanwhile, nearly all female anchors on local and cable news share the news desk with a man—and endure far greater scrutiny for their appearance.

Roles and opportunities in less-serious entertainment media disappear for aging women in a way they don't for men. A classic example is Sally Field (born 1946) playing the love interest of Tom Hanks (born 1956) in the 1988 film *Punchline*, but playing his elderly, dying mother in *Forest Gump* six years later. It is unremarkable for Helen Hunt (born in 1963) to play a romantic lead opposite Jack Nicholson (born in 1937) in *As Good As It Gets*. However, Diane Keaton's "advanced" age (born in 1946) is a central joke of *Something's Gotta Give* when her character becomes Nicholson's romantic interest.

> What is perfection, anyway? It's the death of creativity ...[40]
>
> Diane Keaton

In a scathingly funny 2015 sketch on Comedy Central,[41] Amy Schumer, Tina Fey, Julia Louis-Dreyfus and Patricia Arquette skewer the absurdity of this phenomenon. The four attend a satirical "celebration" of Louis-Dreyfus' "Last F**kable Day," because, she says, "in every actress' life, the media decides when you finally reach the point where you're not believably f**kable anymore." When Schumer naively asks if the same is true for male actors, Arquette replies, "Honey, men don't have that day. Never."

Inside Amy Schumer's head writer Jessi Klein said the sketch came about during a conversation in the writers' room about "actresses aging out of Hollywood and how that happens. Women who were seen as the ultimate hottest ingénue and just like, when do they know? ... Once the phrase 'last f**kable day' came out of someone's mouth ... it became a journey to find the angels who ended up [performing in] it."[42]

Meanwhile, we ridicule women who challenge these realities, celebrate aging, and show more interest in power and fairness than in the power of having fair looks. We mock feminists, lesbians and other "liberated" women for taking such "radical" steps as forgoing make-up and shaved legs. We mock men who wear make-up (unless they are under theatrical lights) or shave their legs (unless they are elite bicycle racers). When we judge an entire gender by its willingness to conform to arbitrary standards, we belittle and disempower all of us.

The logical result of our appearance-based career standards? Historically, women out-earn men in only two professions: modeling and prostitution; "careers" that require practitioners to sell their bodies.

Steps for Aging Beautifully

- Develop a flexible body ideal. Remember that a negative body image is not a necessary side effect of getting older. Age can give you the confidence to create your own unique style.
- Identify with realistic role models. Find older, unglamorous role models who are truly magnificent; and then hold them up as an image with whom to identify. Counteract your own ageism and lookism by trying to see older women as total women.
- Own up to your age. Age acceptance doesn't mean resigning yourself to the stereotype of ageism but redefining those myths as time redesigns your body. If you learn to see yourself in terms of your total assets, not merely in terms of appearance, the "loss" of youthful appearance is balanced by the accomplishments of age.
- Hang on to your sensuality. Indulge your body in all the physical pleasures you've earned by virtue of having lived this long. Keep enjoying the sensual side of movement and keep challenging your body with physical activity.
- Use the wisdom you've acquired over the years. With maturity comes an understanding of what works well for you cosmetically, sexually, athletically, nutritionally. This knowledge can help you nurture your aging body with attention and respect.

Adapted from Rita Freedman's *Bodylove*[43]

Turning the Corner

> If you talked to your friends the way you talk to your body, you'd have no friends left.[44]
>
> Marcia Germaine Hutchinson

If we hope to help ourselves and our children live in healthful ways that foster good relationships, then we have to cast off the pursuit of perfection, and make peace with our bodies. As we saw in Chapter 6, families and loved ones may be willing to change to help support women who are struggling to free themselves from obsessions with weight, food and body image. But the extended family of Western culture reacts cruelly and critically when women try to regain control of their lives and their self-esteem.

I wish our culture's relationship with women reflected the luscious vibrancy in Renoir's paintings of female nudes. Instead, as we've just seen, the picture of women's body image is quite a bit bleaker.

Despite that, women *can* extricate themselves (and one another) from the toxic extended family of commercial media and marketing culture. As we move into chapters exploring treatment and recovery, we'll look at the deeply personal work women must do to make peace with their individual bodies. But we'll also explore the collective efforts we must all make to create a cultural extended family that embraces women as they are, rather than recruiting them to make war on their bodies.

Notes

1 In Caroline Knapp, *Appetites* (New York: Counterpoint, 2002) p. 31.
2 Nacerdine Ouldzeidoune, Joseph Keating, Jane Bertrand and Janet Rice (2013) "A description of female genital mutilation and force-feeding practices in Mauritania: Implications for the protection of child rights and health." *PLoS ONE*, 8 (4): e60594. doi:10.1371/journal.pone.0060594.
3 Gautam Naik, "New obesity boom in Arab countries as old ancestry." *Wall Street Journal*, December 29, 2004. See www.wsj.com/articles/SB110428585970011783 (retrieved August 25, 2015).
4 Robert Durback (Ed.), *Seeds of Hope: A Henri Nouwen Reader* (New York: Image Books, 1997) p.114.
5 Margo Maine, *Body Wars: Making Peace with Women's Bodies* (Carlsbad, CA: Gürze Books, 2000).
6 *Appetites: Why Women Want* (New York: Counterpoint, 2022) p. ix.
7 Viewable at The Barnes Foundation in Philadelphia, Pennsylvania or online at https://en.wikipedia.org/wiki/Pierre-Auguste_Renoir#/media/File:Renoir18.jpg (retrieved August 24, 2105).
8 See also *Bathers*, Barnes Foundation and https://en.wikipedia.org/wiki/Pierre-Auguste_Renoir#/media/File:Pierre_Auguste_Renoir_Les_baigneuses.jpg; and/or *Dance at Bougival*, Boston Museum of Fine Arts and https://en.wikipedia.org/wiki/Pierre-Auguste_Renoir#/media/File:Bougival_Dance.jpg (retrieved August 24, 2015).

9 Claire V. Wiseman, James J. Gray, James E. Mosimann and Anthony H. Ahren (1992) "Cultural expectations of thinness in women: An update." *International Journal of Eating Disorders*, 1 (1), 85–89.

10 Kelly D. Brownell (1991) "Dieting and the search for the perfect body: Where physiology and culture collide." *Behavior Therapy*, 22, 1–12.

11 Nina Bahadur, "It's amazing how much the 'perfect body' has changed in 100 years." *Huffington Post*, posted May 2, 2014. See www.huffingtonpost. com/2014/02/05/perfect-body-change-beauty-ideals_n_4733378.html (retrieved August 24, 2015).

12 "Jag model agency finally puts 'plus-size' & 'straight-size' together." *Huffington Post*, posted July 18, 2013. See www.huffingtonpost.com/2013/07/18/jag-model-agency-plus-size_n_3618630.html (retrieved August 24, 2015).

13 Dhani Mau, "France places ban on too-thin models." *Fashionista*, posted April 3, 2015. See http://fashionista.com/2015/04/france-thin-model-ban-anorexia (retrieved August 24, 2015).

14 1848 quote in Michael S. Kimmel and Thomas E. Mosmiller (Eds.) *Against the Tide: Pro-Feminist Men in the United States, 1776–1990—A Documentary History* (Boston, MA: Beacon Press, 1992) p. xxxi.

15 Ekaterina Walter, "The top 30 stats you need to know when marketing to women." Posted January 24, 2012 on thenextweb.com/ socialmedia/2012/01/24/the-top-30-stats-you-need-to-know-when-marketing-to-women/ (retrieved August 24, 2015).

16 The International Council of Shopping Centers, "Shopping center facts and stats." See www.icsc.org/research/shopping-center-facts-and-stats (retrieved August 24, 2015).

17 Susie Poppick, "More states tax tampons than candy in America." *Money*, posted June 3, 2015. See http://time.com/money/3907775/states-tax-tampons-candy-america/ (retrieved August 24, 2015).

18 See www.whitehouse.gov/equal-pay/myth#top (retrieved May 16, 2015).

19 Katherine Gallagher Robbins and Anne Morrison (2014) "National snapshot: Poverty among women & families, 2013." National Women's Law Center. See www.nwlc.org/sites/default/files/pdfs/povertysnapshot2013.pdf (retrieved August 24, 2015).

20 Transparency Market Research, http://globenewswire.com/news-relea se/2015/01/15/697626/10115697/en/Global-Skincare-Devices-Market-to-Value-US-10-7-Billion-by-2018-Transparency-Market-Research.html#sthash. WiYyktUX.dpuf (retrieved August 24, 2015).

21 In James B. Simpson (Ed.) *Simpson's Contemporary Quotations Since 1950* (Boston, MA: Houghton Mifflin, 1997).

22 eMarketer, "Total US ad spending to see largest increase since 2004" posted July 2, 2014. See www.emarketer.com/Article/Total-US-Ad-Spending-See-Largest-Increase-Since-2004/1010982 (retrieved August 24, 2015).

23 See Jean Kilbourne, *Can't Buy My Love: How Advertising Changes the Way We Think and Feel* (New York: Touchstone, 2000).

24 James B. Twitchell, *Adcult USA: The Triumph of Advertising in American Culture* (New York: Columbia University Press, 1996).

25 Television Bureau of Canada, Inc., "Commercial Lengths." See www.tvb.ca/ pages/commercial+lengths_htm (retrieved August 24, 2015).

26 Scott Donaton & Advertising Age Books, *Madison and Vine: Why the Entertainment and Advertising Industries Must Converge to Survive* (New York: McGraw Hill, 2004).

27 Deborah Then, "Women's magazines: Messages they convey about looks, men, and careers." Paper presented at the annual convention of the American Psychological Association, 1992.

28 *Bossypants* (Boston, MA: Little, Brown and Company, 2013) p. 144.

29 *Madam Secretary* (New York: Miramax, 2005).

30 US Department of Health and Human Services Administration on Aging, "A Profile of older Americans: 2011." See www.aoa.gov/Aging_Statistics/Profile/2011/docs/2011profile.pdf (retrieved August 24, 2015).

31 Ibid.

32 Ari Houser (2007), "Nursing home fact sheet." AARP Public Policy Institute. See http://assets.aarp.org/rgcenter/il/fs10r_homes.pdf (retrieved August 24, 2015).

33 Ibid.

34 Linda Barrett (2014) "Home and community preferences of the 45+ population, 2014." AARP Research Center. See www.aarp.org/content/dam/aarp/research/surveys_statistics/il/2015/2014-Home-Community-45plus-res-il.pdf (retrieved August 24, 2015).

35 Thom File (2014) "Young-adult voting: An analysis of presidential elections, 1964–2012." *Current Population Survey Reports*, pp. 20–572. U.S. Census Bureau, Washington, DC. See www.census.gov/prod/2014pubs/p20-573.pdf (retrieved September 14, 2015).

36 *Moving Beyond Words* (New York: Simon and Schuster, 1994) p. 252.

37 *A Fine Romance* (New York: Simon and Schuster, 2015).

38 Ibid.

39 Bill Carter, "Back talk from 'Murphy Brown' to Dan Quayle," in *The New York Times*, July 20, 1992. See www.nytimes.com/1992/07/20/arts/back-talk-from-murphy-brown-to-dan-quayle.html (retrieved August 24, 2015).

40 *Then Again* (New York: Random House, 2012) p. 193.

41 *Inside Amy Schumer* Season 3, Episode 1; Original air date April 21, 2015, Comedy Central. See www.cc.com/video-clips/a30bcg/inside-amy-schumer-last-f--kable-day---uncensored (retrieved August 24, 2015).

42 Jaimie Etkin, (April 21, 2015). "Tina Fey, Julia Louis-Dreyfus, and Patricia Arquette explain a female actor's 'Last F**kable Day'" *BuzzFeed Entertainment*. See www.buzzfeed.com/jaimieetkin/amy-schumer-tina-fey-julia-louis-dreyfus-patricia-arquette#.nez8A3jD8 (retrieved August 24, 2015).

43 *Bodylove: Learning to Like Our Looks and Ourselves: A Practical Guide for Women—Second Edition* (Carlsbad, CA: Gürze Books, 2002).

44 In Danne Reed, *Fashionably Late: A Sexy Little Twist to Revitalize You and ReDesign Your Life!* (New York: Morgan James Publishing, 2015) p. 29.

8   The Shape of Recovery

So what do you do if it looks or feels like you or a loved one might have an eating disorder or suffer from body image despair?

There is no one simple answer. These multifaceted problems must be addressed from a number of angles, and each woman has to create a unique blend of what works best for her. Much of recovery happens outside formal treatment, when we begin to take chances in life by putting into practice what we learn in therapy. Recovery builds on the willingness to do things differently. Just like love, it is a cluster of small things, not just one "aha."

Women develop eating disorder symptoms as misguided ways to self-soothe. They turn to the eating disorder because they have not learned (or have forgotten) how to calm themselves, handle difficult emotions, or gain a sense of agency and self-worth. Recovery requires finding new and nurturing ways to express and accept the richly imperfect self: the good, the bad and the ugly.

> You are imperfect, permanently and inevitably flawed. And you are beautiful.[1]
>
> Amy Bloom

At first, it may be hard to believe that recovery is possible. Most of my adult patients apologize for needing my time, saying that their problems and the issues underlying their symptoms just aren't important enough. These women have completely absorbed the cultural belief that their true hungers, needs, appetites and feelings are less legitimate and important than their appearance. Listening only to the Voice of Perfection, they are not able to find peace with their bodies.

However, women (and men) can—and do—completely recover from eating disorders, gradually reclaiming their lives, finding their true selves, and accepting their imperfections, frailties and faults.

In the throes of eating disorders and despair over body image, we translate our pain, disappointments and anguish into perfectionist body judgment language (e.g., fat equals failure and worthlessness). In isolation, pain grows like an untreated tumor, spreading, metastasizing, invading and taking over more and more of life. Recovery requires putting feelings into words instead of the perfectionistic language of fat.

> Pain festers in isolation, it thrives in secrecy. Words are its nemesis, naming anguish the first step in defusing it, talking about the muck a woman slogs through—the squirms of self-hatred and guilt, the echoes of emptiness and need—a prerequisite for moving beyond it.[2]
>
> Caroline Knapp

Fortunately, we don't have to do this alone.

Talking about our pain and despair may feel just as frightening as undergoing chemotherapy for cancer—it is strong medicine that might make us feel worse before we feel better. Seeking professional help and finding some safe relationships outside of therapy are both instrumental in the recovery process.

This chapter explores the process of recovery from eating disorder or body image obsessions. These illnesses don't have on/off switches, so recovery is not simple. It requires a process of building motivation and readiness before any change can actually take root. Many women with eating and body image issues get discouraged and give up because they aren't able to make major shifts right away. In reality, no one takes giant steps without taking a lot of baby steps first. Always remember that:

• recovery is possible
• it takes time and effort
• it is not a linear process.

Can Things Change?

Women with eating disorders often wonder if they can survive without their disease because they don't see or feel any separation between the illness and their sense of self. They fear that being symptom-free means they would literally disappear. Some of my patients feel that everyone and everything else in life has let them down or caused too much pain, leaving the eating disorder as their only reliable companion. On the other hand, a woman's eating disorder might mobilize previously unseen (or nonexistent) support and concerns from partners, friends and/or family. Afraid of losing this comfort and attention, she may resist letting go of the problem.

Some women feel hopeless, convinced that they cannot get better because they have been sick for so long. Too afraid to hope, they feel certain that they will fail at recovery—and then feel even worse about themselves. Their hopelessness and ambivalence are self-protective. Others believe they deserve to be punished and that God (or some other Power) will not allow them to be happy or feel better.

Patients who are skeptical or ambivalent about recovery frequently say these things to me:

- What if I work really hard at getting better and I still die? I don't want to die and I especially don't want to be fat. Will it be worth it?
- I don't deserve to feel better. I have messed up my life and have no one else to blame. This is my punishment.
- Nothing has ever worked out for me, why should I believe I can get better?
- If I give up my eating disorder but don't feel any better, then what will I have?

This ambivalence and despair are powerful, and fueled by the obsession's self-defeating Voice of Perfection. Meanwhile, malnutrition's impact on brain neurotransmitters causes depression. (People who binge and/or purge *and* people who restrict suffer from malnutrition stemming from poor nutritional intake, independent of how much they eat or weigh.) Together, these factors can make it feel nearly impossible to take the leap of faith necessary to begin recovery.

There is no denying that recovery from these illnesses is hard work, requiring major changes in how we think, feel and live. Many women who have recovered found it helps to break down recovery into these smaller pieces or stages.

- **Contemplating change:** I'm aware there is a problem. I'm waiting until later to do anything, or I feel ambivalent about whether to do anything.
- **Preparing for change:** I'm getting ready to do something soon, or I recently began to try some new attitudes and behaviors.
- **Taking action:** I'm working to overcome the problem by actively altering my behavior, self-perceptions, beliefs and/or my surrounding environment.
- **Preserving change:** I'm taking steps and getting support to prevent relapses, and maintain my new positive, healthy life pattern.[3]

Looking at things this way, we can see ambivalence as an important *part* of recovery. Vacillation is a stage of change rather than a stubborn resistance to it. We also recognize that maintenance of recovery is a process of ongoing change and growth. We realize that the road of recovery is a healthy journey, not another pursuit of perfection. It comes with surprises and new challenges.

There is no problem that doesn't have within it the seeds for its solution.[4]

Alexandra Stoddard

Readiness for Change

If you are struggling with issues about eating or body image, this exercise can help clarify your next steps. In each group of statements, check the one (or ones) that best describe where you are right now.

Group 1
☐ **A** I don't think there's anything wrong with how I feel about food or my body.
☐ **B** I need to do something different; this really isn't working for me.
☐ **C** I'm going to do something about this soon.
☐ **D** Reading fashion magazines makes me feel worse about myself; I'm giving them up.

Group 2
☐ **A** Other people badger me about this; they don't know what they're talking about.
☐ **B** When I'm ready, I'll be able to do something about this.
☐ **C** I am discussing this problem with my partner, friend, or doctor.
☐ **D** I am starting to eat regular meals every day.

Group 3
☐ **A** It's normal to obsess about weight and food, and not be able to think about anything else.
☐ **B** I am afraid others will think less of me if I gain weight or look different.
☐ **C** I'm going to get professional help; I can't do this alone.
☐ **D** I won't buy any more fat-free or binge foods (or diet pills, laxatives, etc.).

Group 4
☐ **A** I'm fine; other people are just jealous of my self-control.
☐ **B** I'd like to be able to order off the menu without making any changes.
☐ **C** I'll read the self-help book that helped my friend.
☐ **D** I am throwing the scale out.

Group 5
☐ **A** Exercise is more important than having friends.
☐ **B** I'd like to be able to have more balance in my life.
☐ **C** My New Years' resolution will be to eat better.
☐ **D** I'm posting positive affirmations on my mirror so I won't be as negative about my body.

A answers indicate you are in the pre-contemplation stage, not sure that there's anything wrong.
B answers indicate that you are contemplating making some changes but haven't quite started yet.
C answers are signs that you are preparing to change.
D answers indicate that you have already started to take action.

If you have a mixture of responses, you are moving from one stage to the next. Ambivalence about change is common. Motivation to change is not a yes/no thing—it evolves. Even reading this book could be the beginning of a change process!

The Shape of Treatment

A serious eating disorder or body image obsession affects all dimensions of the sufferer's life—identity, spirituality, relationships, work, family— and every biological system in the body itself. Effective treatment uses multiple strategies to address these disparate elements together, rather than approaching them individually, in isolation.

- An individual session with a *psychologist* may include conversations about emotions, family, medical issues and the sufferer's relationship to her body and to food.
- Consultations with a *physician* might include discussions of emotional struggles, nutrition and pressing medical concerns.
- Discussions with a *dietitian* may explore family history of food related issues, work environment and meals.

Eating disorders expert Dr. Anita Johnston, author of *Eating In the Light of the Moon*, describes the treatment process as a labyrinth: a single pathway that often loops back toward itself while moving forward at the same time. She writes that women working their way through recovery:

> follow a twisting, turning, winding path to their centers … to leave behind old perceptions of themselves that they had adopted from others and to reclaim their inner authorities … to listen to the voice from within to give them guidance and support as they searched for their true thoughts, feelings and desires …letting go of all expectations of linear progress, disengaging the rational mind, and embracing the power of their emotions and intuition.[5]

Recovery's leap of faith eventually blossoms into a willingness to explore new places in ourselves, our relationships and our world. Some steps on the journey are slow and tentative, others come more easily—but each can be taken only one step at a time.

Recovery Isn't a Race

When beginning treatment, most of my patients ask, "How long will this take?" Despite decades treating women with eating disorders and body image problems, it is impossible to answer that question. No matter how wise or experienced, a professional can never predict precisely how long it will take a particular woman to recover from her particular crisis. An orthopedist can predict that your broken leg will heal in about six weeks, but eating disorders are exponentially more complex than bone fractures. This truism often frustrates clients and families. Clinicians share this frustration—but the lack of perfect predictability is simply in the nature of eating disorders. In addition, each woman is different, no matter how similar her symptoms or problem behaviors may be to those of other women.

As long as we look at recovery as a continuum, rather than a single destination or a cure, there is plenty of reason to hope and to anticipate how we can actually improve our lives. Even if we've been struggling for years, we can become less tormented and grow healthier. It helps to give up old either/or reasoning that equates self-worth or goodness only with perfection.

In the end, it is crucial to remember that, like life itself, recovery isn't a race. Recovery is progress, not perfection, and the only formula that holds the real promise of peace.

Recovery is hindered when we *judge* ourselves harshly by what we can see of someone else's journey. We can't know what goes on inside others, and even understanding our own problems is a challenge. On the other hand, a healthy *comparison* with someone doing well in recovery can inspire us to see that recovery is possible. Remember that if we have suffered for years (or even decades), we won't get better with just a handful of therapy sessions, visits to the doctor, or consultations with a nutritionist. And treatment alone won't do it—what we do outside of treatment matters, too. Change does not come instantly. As a wise woman once told me, "A tincture of time is the best medicine."

Some of my former clients simply did not believe they could ever change how they saw themselves or treated their bodies. After entering treatment, however, they allowed themselves to hope instead of be hopeless, to share their stories and their pain instead of isolating themselves, and to rely on other human beings for help instead of continuing their lonely Superwoman stance of needing no one. They stopped listening to the Voice of Perfection, or at least turned down the volume.

Still at war with women's bodies, the larger culture provides little positive support for recovery. While we can't change our culture overnight, we can change our reaction to it and learn to take better care of ourselves. I never promise new patients that they are going to feel great about their bodies, even though some do eventually embrace their bodies fully. But even the women who remain occasionally haunted by perfectionism *can* find ways to tune in to more positive voices, and focus on other, more important pleasures in life.

If in the past you had a negative treatment experience or just feel it didn't help, try again. You may be more ready now, at a different point in your life. It may be that a new and different approach will work better for you. Try to have Beginner's Mind (see more later and in Chapter 10) and be open to what is possible now that may not have worked for you in the past.

How Does It Work?

The length and progression of treatment depend on the patient and the professionals. At the minimum, an adult woman with eating or body image disorders needs an individual therapist experienced in eating disorders, body image and women's health to assess the situation and recommend the continuum of care she needs. Usually, *individual therapy* is vital to the ongoing process of treatment, because it helps uncover the deeper issues below the symptoms. In this one-on-one therapeutic relationship, a woman gets understanding and support as she takes the brave steps toward change, gradually removes the mask of perfection, and learns to be her true self. As she gains confidence in the safe confines of therapy, she grows more assured in her other relationships. A skilled therapist also helps a patient to begin changing her behaviors, set reasonable goals, and work through the anxiety engendered by giving up old habits.

Finding the Right Help

The cornerstone of treatment for eating disorders is developing a trusting relationship with a primary therapist—the person we work with most closely. Usually this is a trusted individual therapist, specializing in eating and body image issues, who can direct us to other necessary services. Of course, we can't measure trust on a scale—it is a feeling. Still there are some guidelines to use to find that person.

First, ask for recommendations from friends who have had similar experiences, a medical provider, or other professionals you trust (clergy, nurses, social workers). You can also find resources on the Internet, or from local mental health associations and hospitals. (We list some resources in the Appendix.)

Once you have some therapists' names, call (or visit the therapist's website) and ask for basic information such as:

- Are you a specialist in eating and body image problems?
- How long have you specialized in this area?
- What other problems do you treat?
- What degrees and licenses do you have?
- What are your fees? How do you handle payments and insurance reimbursement?
- What is the availability of appointments?
- What is your evaluation process?
- Will you need any medical information prior to my appointment?
- How do you develop a treatment plan and how do we know if it is working?
- What is your treatment approach or philosophy?
- Are you comfortable working with physicians, dietitians and other potential members of my treatment team?
- What form of family involvement should I expect?

The first appointment should be an evaluation on both sides. It helps to talk about your motivation for treatment, what you tried in the past, and how successful those past efforts were. You both should discuss treatment options and other forms of therapy that might help. Openly discuss how you both will evaluate progress, determine whether a different level of care is needed, and what to expect in terms of the course and duration of treatment.

After the first session, reflect on the following questions and answer them honestly.

- How do I feel about the therapist and the surroundings?
- What is my comfort level?
- If I'm uncomfortable, is it due to the therapist? Or is it due to the feelings stirred up by seeking help and being honest about my behaviors and emotions?

A good individual therapist can help us decide how and when to include other family members. Sometimes arranging *marital* or *family therapy* with a separate professional is best, so that we can keep dedicated attention on our own personal growth in individual therapy. In other cases, we may be able to integrate our spouse, partner, children, or other family members into periodic sessions with our individual therapist. One way or another, marital and family sessions help break negative patterns that keep us stuck in unhealthy relationships with food and our body. They also help our partner and family understand what we are dealing with and how best to support us.

Being in *group therapy* with other women facing body image and eating problems can dramatically decrease a woman's sense that no one really understands, or that others will judge and condemn her. It is easier to take risks when we see our peers doing the same and we can draw strength from their shared experiences and successes. In addition, group therapy invites us to recognize and respond—with clarity and compassion—to other participants' struggles and symptom behaviors, a practice which promotes clarity and compassion toward our own situation. Group therapy can also provide the joy and life-altering comfort of noncompetitive relationships with other women.

However, group therapy also has the potential to accentuate negative competitive behaviors (who's thinnest, sickest, or exercises the most?), so it's important to be in a professionally led group and to talk regularly with one's primary therapist about whether the group is actually helping.

Nutritional counseling is essential for most people in eating disorders recovery, and very useful for addressing body image issues. It also improves food intake and balance, while challenging misinformation or mistaken beliefs about food. It is easier to make major changes in how and what we eat when we understand the true physical and health consequences of those decisions.

Many registered dietitians focus on weight loss and managing chronic diseases—and do not have the specialized skills and knowledge to deal with eating disorders. So, if a dietitian's waiting room or website materials emphasize weight management and BMI, she or he may not be best for you.

Finding a dietitian or nutritionist specifically trained in problems resulting from disordered eating may take extra effort, but it's essential. She or he will assess your nutritional intake and can quickly identify areas where it is deficient—and how those deficiencies keep your eating disorder going. Many of my adult patients eat —they just don't eat enough, they eat things that don't sustain them, they binge and purge, or they burn up nutrition too quickly through excess exercise. These behavior patterns keep their lives and bodies focused on food (another demonstration of how the body instinctively defends itself against starvation). While dietary counseling alone is seldom enough to change these behaviors, it can increase your motivation, provide accurate information about your nutritional needs, correct some of your misguided beliefs about food, and reduce fears about making changes.

Body image, movement and creative arts therapies use a variety of experiential approaches to help heal the conflict between body image and self-image. Talking therapies are essential, but therapeutic body movement and art expression can profoundly alter old patterns, perceptions, feelings and bodily sensations.[6] This helps us be and feel more connected to our bodies, and to find a new way to relate to ourselves and others. Most specialized eating disorders treatment programs include art and/or movement therapy, but it can be difficult to find these services outside of a formal program.

Medical treatment is a critical component of recovery. Women need early and regular medical evaluations to find out if any of the symptoms stem from underlying diseases like malignancies, chronic infections, diabetes, thyroid disorders, kidney dysfunction, or inflammatory bowel diseases. When the overall treatment process begins, an assessment of how our eating or body disorders have affected the body's systems and organs will determine the level of immediate medical care necessary. Minimally, an electrocardiogram and blood work should be done at the outset of treatment (and regularly thereafter) to prevent life-threatening heart attacks or other potentially debilitating problems. The therapist, dietitian and medical provider must collaborate regularly to assess any immediate physiological danger.

Psychiatric medications help some women during the course of recovery. When appropriately prescribed and monitored, antidepressants can often help control compulsive behaviors and mood, especially early in treatment, when changing behaviors is so unsettling. Antianxiety or sleep medications are sometimes prescribed, but in many cases, improved nutrition does more than any drug to improve the mood, anxiety and sleep disorders that accompany eating problems and poor nutrition. So it is wise to give careful consideration to what (if any) medications are used as tools in recovery.

Western medicine has a history of excessively medicating women. Because it is cheaper and less time-consuming to medicate eating and body disorders than it is to treat them comprehensively, our health care system often pressures physicians to provide prescriptions (with little or no monitoring of their effectiveness) rather than to provide the multifaceted therapy necessary for recovery. The bottom line: psychiatric medication alone can't fix eating and body disorders.

We must take an active part in decisions about all aspects of our treatment, whether medical, nutritional, or psychological. The insights gained through therapy and the resultant changed perceptions of self, relationships and the world are the most important tools for making progress in recovery.

Spiritual growth supports and weaves through all aspects of recovery. Many women struggling with body and eating disorders say they don't rely on spiritual beliefs or support systems. To recover, we must nurture our faith that things can change for the better, trust in our professional helpers, hope for the future and believe that there is more to life than the body. If we don't believe, relief won't come. Spiritual growth can come from formal religious traditions or from less organized forms of faith. We all have spirituality that (like our physical health) needs attention and nurturance to make it work for us the best it can.

Many who recover from eating and body image obsessions are drawn to a *political and cultural awareness* about the role women play in society and the negative messages about body issues we continually receive. This consciousness gives a larger context for why we battle our bodies so severely. This helps us feel less sick or crazy, and is an important tool as we choose recovery instead of our culture's perfectionistic and unreachable images of women.

In her recovery, Jennifer began finding her voice and feeling more personal power when she started lobbying against websites that glorified eating disorders. Although these websites didn't contribute directly to her illness, she understood how they endorsed and encouraged extremely unhealthy behaviors that endanger others. After recovering from bulimia, Louise started a foundation to help women access eating disorders treatment. Becoming an activist was critical to her recovery and makes her feel that something positive is resulting from her years of pain.

Treatment Philosophy

Therapists and treatment programs tend to emphasize one or more ways of conceptualizing eating and body image disorders, and this section briefly describes the most common viewpoints.[7] It is important to ask therapists what underlying philosophy or philosophies guide their work. These various models can be, and often are, integrated. For example, my therapeutic approach is primarily a feminist relational model. After working for years in a hospital-based treatment program, I am also very familiar with the medical model. I can draw on therapeutic tools from my training and experience in family therapy, my knowledge of 12-step programs, and my familiarity with psychodynamic theory, object relations and attachment theory, as well as cognitive and behavioral treatment principles. Experienced eating disorders therapists often develop similar levels of eclectic knowledge.

In general I recommend that women struggling with concerns about eating and body image work with therapists and programs that respect the tenets of feminist theory, and acknowledge the unique pressures on women in today's culture. This does not rule out working with a male therapist—men can be feminists and male therapists working in this field usually are.

The Medical Model: The Body is Sick

The Medical Model focuses on the body itself and measures treatment progress by weight goals, eating correctly, and controlling symptomatic behaviors. The Medical Model usually pays little attention to the patient's underlying issues or how she experiences the treatment. Medical intervention is essential in order to get an acutely ill patient out of danger, but as treatment proceeds, the medical model alone has limited effectiveness in treating eating disorders.

The Behavioral Model: The Behavior is Sick

The behavioral approach also focuses on the symptoms rather than on the underlying issues. A strict behavioral approach manages symptoms with rewards and punishments for progress and problems. This was a common eating disorders treatment model in the past, but it did not prove effective over the long term. It may even be harmful when used as the only approach. When a woman feels forced to change a behavior too quickly, she may regress, or else develop new disordered behaviors to cope with the stress. For example, if a woman with anorexia is pressured to gain weight without exploring and understanding the reasons for her food obsession, she may put on the pounds but then begin purging for the first time to relieve her unaddressed emotional disturbances. In the same way, if a woman with binge eating disorder is pressured to diet and lose weight—without addressing why she developed BED—she may be caught in a spiral of weight loss and weight gain that wreaks havoc on her health and self-esteem.

The Cognitive Model: The Thoughts are Sick

Instead of focusing on behavior, the Cognitive Model attempts to redirect and reshape the thoughts that initiate and support the eating disorder or body image obsession. This systematic approach is often used in group therapy and can be found in printed manuals and online treatment packages. The Cognitive Model identifies and then challenges maladaptive beliefs and thoughts, on the theory that this will in turn change the maladaptive behavior.

The Addiction Model: The Woman is Sick

Eating and body image obsessions share some similarities with addictions like alcoholism, but there are some important differences too (see p. 150). Some aspects of eating disorders are addictive, like the physical dependence on laxatives or diuretics described in Chapter 5. Both illnesses share frequent denial, the need to hit bottom before seeing the need to get help, powerlessness over the problem behavior, the possibility of relapse and the need to grow spiritually in recovery.

The Family Systems Model: The Family is Sick

This model is built on understanding how family dynamics can help create and feed psychological problems. Family systems therapy targets interactions, boundaries and multigenerational patterns within families. The philosophy is that improving family system patterns will enable the person with symptoms to stop her harmful behaviors and achieve recovery.

The Feminist Model: Cultural Expectations for Women and Our Appearance are Sick

Like the Family Systems Model, the Feminist Model does not believe that eating disorders and body image despair are rooted exclusively in the individual. It takes a more cultural and global view, seeing eating and body image behaviors as coping mechanisms that women of all ages use to deal with sexism, racism, weightism, lookism, consumerism, sexual abuse and other forces—like the pressures to be perfect—that harm and limit female lives. While other models tend to place the therapist in the role of expert, the feminist approach encourages a partnership between therapist and client, setting mutual goals, and helping the client to find healthier ways to relate to herself, others and the larger world.

Where is Treatment?

Body image and eating disorders treatment programs operate in a number of different physical settings, which work best when matched properly with the severity of current symptoms. Unfortunately, the final decision is often determined by the sufferer's insurance coverage and ability to pay, rather than by which resources are most effective for the particular patient.

Outpatient treatment works best for someone who is medically stable, has an adequate support system, and is motivated to work on problems while continuing to live at home and function normally at work, home and socially. It may consist of separate appointments for individual, family, or group therapy, along with nutritional counseling; or it may be an intensive outpatient program blending these services together through sessions in the evenings and/or on weekends.

Inpatient treatment takes place in a hospital or medical center. It is generally used for patients who need acute medical facilities nearby. These people are physiologically unstable (with depressed or fluctuating vital signs, very low weight or significant weight fluctuations, electrolyte imbalance, complications from other illnesses such as diabetes, and the like) or psychiatrically unstable (with rapidly worsening symptoms, severe symptoms that aren't yet responsive to other treatment, suicide risk, and the like).

In *residential treatment*, patients live at a facility dedicated exclusively to eating disorders recovery. Residential programs are usually not in a hospital building, although some are housed on hospital grounds. This setting is suitable for patients who are psychiatrically unable to respond to partial hospital or outpatient treatment, but are physiologically stable enough to go without daily acute or intensive medical care.

In *partial hospital* programs, patients are treated for many hours a day inside an outpatient treatment center or hospital, but then return home in the evening. Partial hospitalization works for patients who still need daily monitoring of their medical status (but are not at immediate risk) and who are psychiatrically impaired (unable to function in their normal daily roles and/or still engage in their symptoms daily). This setting provides intensive treatment, which the person gets to take home and practice for a few hours before returning for the next day's intensive therapy.

Eating and body image issues pose particular challenges to the traditional *self-help recovery* model. These challenges are not well understood by many well-meaning people who, for example, expect the 12 steps of Alcoholics Anonymous to transfer easily to the treatment of eating disorders. Such notions are understandable, since eating disorders share many similarities with addiction. But the differences between the two types of illness are profound, making it potentially dangerous to use 12-step recovery tools on eating disorders without the guidance of treatment professionals or Eating Disorders Anonymous (EDA).

Recovery from drug or alcohol addiction requires wrenching changes in the addict's every relationship, routine and habit. People with eating disorders must make similar changes in order to achieve recovery. But an addict's body won't die if she completely abstains from drugs or alcohol. On the other hand, no one's body can survive chronic malnourishment or complete abstinence from food. There is no healthy escape from our daily physical need to eat, or the necessity of living every moment inside our bodies. Since abstinence isn't a recovery option for eating and body image disorders, we have to find other ways to make peace with our body, body image and food.

EDA was founded to integrate the strengths of 12-step programs and the unique needs of people with eating disorders.

> In EDA, recovery means living without obsessing on food, weight and body image. In our eating disorders, we sometimes felt like helpless victims. Recovery means gaining or regaining the power to see our options, to make careful choices in our lives. Recovery means rebuilding trust with ourselves, a gradual process that requires much motivation and support. As we learn and practice careful self-honesty, self-care and self-expression, we gain authenticity, perspective, peace and empowerment.[8]

The most basic difference between EDA and other 12-step programs is the approach to abstinence. Abstinence from chemical use is the core of drug and alcohol addiction *treatment*, but abstinence from food (or a desire to be abstinent that leads to bingeing) lies at the core of many eating disorder *symptoms*.

Programs built on the 12 steps help millions of people overcome addictive behavior and regain their health. Wisely, EDA makes the subtle and important shift away from AA's traditional concepts of abstinence.

Some eating and body disorder treatment programs also incorporate 12-step practices but change the language to reflect the realities of eating disorders.[9]

Take AA's first step, which reads "We admitted we were powerless over alcohol—that our lives had become unmanageable." A woman with an eating disorder would have to reframe and reword that step for it to help her recovery. Instead of admitting that she is powerless over the *external* substance of food, she would find the source of her powerlessness in her *internal* qualities like perfectionism, a tendency to take care of others before herself, or constant self-shaming. Thus, instead of abstaining from food, she would strive to abstain from the negative ways she treats herself. In a sense, women with eating and body disorders are addicted to how they see and treat themselves, more than to the external elements of the illness.

Overeaters Anonymous, a 12-step fellowship for people struggling with compulsive overeating, may seem like a logical place to get support for eating and body image problems. However, some of OA's focus on eating may reinforce dangerous good food–bad food dichotomous thinking that supports eating disorders. OA's fellowship, with its physical, emotional and spiritual approach, helps some people with eating disorders. However, I recommend EDA as an alternative. In the end, if 12-step programs have helped you with past life problems, work with a therapist to develop healthy ways of integrating those principles into your journey of recovery from food and body disorders.

Obstacles to Getting Help

Ambivalence, denial and the stubbornness of eating and body image disorders are not the only barriers to recovery. Insurance often covers mental health very differently from the way it covers physical health, and that can be a rude awakening for someone seeking help.

Although eating disorders are the most lethal psychiatric illness they are still poorly understood. As a result, many people have to fight their insurance companies for adequate treatment. If your insurance comes through a large employer, I suggest going to the human resources department, union, or whoever ultimately holds the contract with your insurance company to request help in advocating for your teatment and recovery. When an insurance company stands to lose a contract, it may suddenly find ways to be flexible.

Most women who recover from these disorders had to fight hard to obtain the treatment that addressed their particular needs. One woman who succeeded in getting coverage says, "When someone at the insurance company says no, assume that he's really saying 'I don't know,' and don't stop asking until you hear a yes you can use." The person saying no usually knows little or nothing about your actual condition. The "no" is more about corporate profits than about what you need—it does not mean that you are not sick, or that you don't "deserve" treatment.

Strong advocacy has persuaded some insurance companies to pool mental health and medical benefits to cover necessary treatment. After being denied coverage or care, some women have hired lawyers, recruited state attorneys general and lobbied legislators to challenge the inequity. In the meantime, we have to get help anyway we can. This takes a fair amount of energy, but it can be a good job for a family member, especially someone who struggles with knowing how else to help.

My website (www.pressuretobeperfect.com) has suggestions for fighting the system and getting help. The National Eating Disorders Association (NEDA) has strategies, fact sheets, sample letters and other resources online at www.nationaleatingdisorders.org/insurance-resources—including research citations that document the proven benefits of proper care.[10]

In the meantime, many professionals and families have banded together to fight for better coverage for eating disorders. After all, eating disorders and body image obsessions now represent a major public health problem, primarily affecting women, which should have major federal recognition and support. The Eating Disorders Coalition for Research, Policy, and Action (www.eatingdisorderscoalition.org) advocates the US Government for treatment resources; access to treatment; and funding for research, education and prevention. Meanwhile, NEDA lobbies at federal, state and local levels for the same aims. Both EDC and NEDA hold regular "lobby days" where recovered people and family members meet with legislators and policymakers. Participating in advocacy activities can help you and other people at the same time.

New Ways to Shape Your Thinking

While there is no one way to achieve recovery, some universals do exist, such as the need to avoid self-blame and the importance of changing distorted thinking about our body, weight and food.

Eating and body obsessions don't follow an A-causes-B-causes-C kind of pattern with simple, clear conclusions. We have to accept that we will never understand everything that led to an eating or body obsession. Instead it helps to imagine our life and problems as one of those "connect-the dots" children's puzzles. Connecting two dots doesn't solve the puzzle, but the more dots we connect, the more sense we can make of the total picture.

I urge my patients to appreciate that their complicated behaviors start out as survival techniques, serving as a life preserver. At a gut level, my patients felt that they would drown if they let go of the symptom behaviors. Instead of berating ourselves for using an obsession to stay afloat, we can learn how it functioned in our life—and then release it as we build sturdy new ships to sail healthfully through our future.

As women enter and work through recovery, they rely on those who have gone before them to help show the way. Below are short descriptions of some common steps other women have taken in achieving and maintaining recovery.

All suffering is bearable if it is seen as part of a story.[11]

Isak Dinesen

Develop your life story. Acknowledge the people and events that shaped your life, both positively and negatively. Discover how often or seldom you met your real needs and hungers, and how that relates to obsessions about weight, food and body image. As you come to understand your life story, you will naturally become less critical and harsh with yourself; you may even learn to empathize with yourself. This, in turn, will make you less likely to think negative and self-blaming thoughts that open the gates for the self-punitive behaviors of bingeing, restricting, over-exercising, or purging.

Add up the balance sheet. In addition to understanding how eating and body obsessions functioned as flawed life preservers, begin to explore the price you paid for using them. When you felt good about controlling what you ate, was there anything else you truly enjoyed about your life? What was the quality of your relationships with others? These obsessions always take us away from real people and real pleasure. As you progress through recovery, relapse looks less attractive when you periodically reflect on such questions.

Even a stopped clock is right twice a day.[12]

Catherine Hughes Barnes

Self-knowledge never ends. There are many paths to insight. Never a fixed state or end-product, insight is an ongoing process of self-awareness that grows richer and deeper as you proceed. Continued individual therapy can help uncover ongoing insights. Family therapy or informal discussions with family members can help uncover family secrets and patterns that give context to your experience. Group therapy can uncover new understanding about your own experience as you and your peers share life stories, strategies and future hopes.

Make time to reflect. We can't develop insight or nurture ourselves if we maintain "perfect" Superwoman schedules that leave no time to reflect or process our experience. Rather than keeping busy to avoid thinking about the shape you're in, reserve daily time to stop moving, sit down, and be quiet with yourself through meditation, journaling, or other self-awareness strategies. Journaling can be a great way to develop a deeper appreciation of your goodness and foster insight into (and appreciation for) your imperfections. When you allow yourself to write down perceptions without filtering and critique, you learn a great deal. The more frequently you make time for reflection, the more helpful it will be.

Time is the mother of perspective.[13]

Judith Hayes

Remember that fat is not a feeling; it is a shorthand code word for a much more complicated emotional state. Whenever that three-letter *f* word comes up in conversation or drifts into your mind, use it as a signal to dig deeper and find out what you are really feeling in that moment (journaling can help a lot with this). It might be sadness, anxiety, fear, loss, inadequacy, loneliness, shame, or other difficult emotions. Our culture teaches women that their feelings are not important or legitimate, so fat becomes the code word to describe any and all negative or painful feelings. It is hard to stop speaking the language of fat, and figure out all these complicated feelings. But the insights and rewards are great when you move out of your head and into your heart to trust your gut feelings and intuition.

We usually feel worse before we feel better. For years, your eating or body disorder masked and numbed feelings of pain and joy. When the symptoms start to fade, you will feel emotions more intensely than you have in ages. You may address certain life issues head-on for the first time. It will not be easy, but the painful feelings will not last forever. All feelings pass, so cherish the good ones when they are present and recall them fondly when they go. Meanwhile, remember that the difficult emotions also flow away if you let them.

Time has passed through me and become a song.[14]

Holly Near

Now is the only time you have. Planning how you're going to feel next week is a waste of time and energy—plus it may keep you from realizing it when you *actually do* feel better. Instead, work on developing what Buddhists call "Beginner's Mind," allowing life to happen in the moment rather than trying to predict (perfectly) every permutation of the unknowable future.

In the beginner's mind there are many possibilities, but in the expert's mind there are few.[15]

Jon Kabat-Zinn

Practice being less of an expert and more of a participant in your life. This requires relinquishing the pursuit of perfection, an important ingredient in recovery that brings many other rewards.

Never fear feelings. Covering up emotions does much more harm than meeting them head-on. Louise, whose severe eating disorder controlled her life for more than twenty years, says she binged to get away from bad feelings, and then purged because she felt bad about the bingeing. This led to feeling bad about her purging, which she avoided by bingeing again. This vicious, destructive cycle spun on the avoidance of other bad feelings that Louise eventually had to confront anyway to recover. She says:

> The pain of my eating disorder was measurable; I knew what it would be. It was my system to keep me safe. I was scared of everything else. I thought all those bad feelings would be too much for me. It turns out I was wrong. I went through treatment more than once and had to face up to those emotions. I would want to run away again, and sometimes I did. But in the end, those feelings didn't kill me, or even keep on hurting me. I survived, and now, for the first time, I get to really experience the good feelings too, because they got pushed down and away just as much as my bad feelings did.

Louise used her eating disorder like a cocoon to separate herself from difficult emotions and problems. In recovery, she learned to cope with tough feelings and challenges by breaking them down into what she had to face in the here and now. Frequently, my advice to patients is to just deal with "what's in your face." We don't have to solve all of our problems at once.

Respect the shadow. Everyone has angry, brooding thoughts and feelings. Don't fear or judge them. Because women are taught the myth that aggression and anger are not feminine, we tend to reject these very natural feelings, and criticize ourselves for having them.

If harnessed wisely, powerful feelings like anger can be creative, constructive, and transforming. Rosa Parks was angry about being ordered to give up her seat to a white man on a Montgomery, Alabama bus in 1955. Her refusal is an iconic moment in the civil rights movement, which gradually challenged and transformed race relations in the United States. Consider Mothers Against Drunk Driving. Founded by *women* hurt and *angry* about intoxicated drivers killing their children, MADD changed laws and increased conviction rates nationwide. Even the group's name, MADD, is a powerful example of constructive anger in the service of love. Let your shadow of angry feelings work for you instead of against you.

> We wish to make rage into a fire that cooks things rather than a fire of conflagration.[16]
>
> Clarissa Pinkola Estés

Recognize and trust appetites. Our culture confuses women about their appetites, teaching that calories and fat grams are more important than joy and passion. Taught to want a constricted body instead of a full spirit, our intuitive sense of our needs and hungers begins to fade. Figuring out what you really want becomes a dumbfounding challenge. The next time you feel a food binge or a shopping frenzy coming on, stop and ask: What am I really hungry for? The question may be harder to answer than you imagine, but the answer is what will truly satisfy your appetite for living.

Adjust Your Aging Attitudes. There is no denying that growing older means losing your youth, but these years can also bring a gradual liberation from youth's dependency on others' opinions and approval (with all the concerns about how others see us). Mark Twain wisely observed that, in his youth, he worried continually about what people thought about him, but when he got older, he realized that nobody was thinking about him—they were busy thinking about themselves! Letting go appears to be the mantra of healthy and happy folks who thrive as they age. Adopting an attitude that embraces the feelings and experience of being alive can replace the old control junkie, and make you a lot happier.

As we age, many of us have more influence at work and in our communities. We may have more disposable income to support good causes, pursue our hobbies, travel, and enjoy other well-earned pleasures. With better medical treatment and disease prevention, we are more likely to live longer and to stay well. With good health and less pressure to prove ourselves, we may find renewed energy for relationships, personal challenge, spirituality, renewal and contentment.

Some women enter politics or start their own businesses at midlife, tapping renewed sources of ambition and aggression. Since we have less estrogen and more testosterone, we can blend the masculine and feminine in new ways. We may even get comfortable being seen as different or a little eccentric, welcoming comparison to a grandmother or aunt who was seen as a character, complete with odd habits and gray hair.

> I don't have great thighs. I have great big breasts and a soft little tummy; glam Jamie, the perfect Jamie is such a fraud. The more I like me, the less I want to pretend to be other people.[17]
>
> Jamie Lee Curtis

Make relationships feed you. Many women develop patterns of selflessness in intimate relationships, which leaves them hungry for their own needs to be met. You may worry that others won't like you anymore if you presume to meet your needs, and not just theirs. While you may think this approach makes you an expert on what others feel, it actually leaves you feeling incomplete, alone, misunderstood, and hungry for more. A relationship is pretty shallow if only one person's needs are being met.

On the recovery journey, you must tune in to your feelings and needs, paying at least as much attention to your needs as you do to the other person's. You can be assertive, ask for what you want, and say how you other: perfection/failure, thin/fat, in control/out of control. When it comes to the body, they know how to judge and deprive themselves. They know how to do too much, but not how to act in moderation.

Because we are human, we will make mistakes. If we believe every mistake is a total failure, then we inevitably believe that we will continue failing forever. This is a recipe for hopelessness and unhealthy behavior, rather than for growth and progress. Dichotomous thinking also makes us fear *success* because it represents a radical change and departure from the safety and predictability of what we know—even if all we let ourselves know is failure. We lose a lot by staying in a dichotomous world—it may seem safe, but it is really very dangerous.

Changing entrenched patterns of dichotomous reasoning takes practice, but it opens the door to self-forgiveness, patience and an appreciation that life (and recovery) is a process. More realistic reasoning brings awareness but not always immediate changes in our behavior or symptoms. It is always easier to have an insight than to change behavior. New self-knowledge may even set our behavior back a bit as we process the information before moving forward again. We must be patient with ourselves, even if our patience only lasts ten minutes. The best approach to recovery is one day at a time, sometimes one hour at a time or one meal at a time, just putting one foot in front of the other, and doing the next right, healthy thing.

> You need to learn how to select your thoughts just the same way you select your clothes every day. This is a power you can cultivate. If you want to control things in your life so bad, work on the mind. That's the only thing you should be trying to control.[2]
>
> Elizabeth Gilbert

Restructuring Cognitive Distortion

Rigid either/or reasoning is deeply intertwined with The Voice of eating and body image disorders we discussed in Chapter 5. The Voice and dichotomous reasoning keep us feeling bad all the time—these *cognitive distortions* cause real pain and suffering. Below are cognitive distortions known to fuel eating disorders and body image obsessions.

- Personalization: We blame ourselves for things that are not our fault, take everything too personally, and see ourselves as responsible for things that have nothing to do with us.
- Terminal uniqueness: We think that no one else has or can understand our problems and situation. We believe that we are all alone and doomed to stay that way.
- Dichotomous thinking: Everything we see and experience is either black or white, all or nothing. For example, we only see ourselves as perfect or worthless, fat or thin.

feel. You can choose relationships wisely, spending more time with friends who help you to feel good about yourself and little (or no) time with people who put you down or bring out your sense of competition and negativity. You can have intimate friendships with other women that don't include competing over weight, dieting, appearance, or anything else.

Getting a Journal Started

As long as a journal makes sense to you, it has accomplished its goal. You don't have to worry about sentence structure, punctuation, or legibility. So let go of any hang-ups you have about writing; this is therapy, not school!

- Set aside ten minutes each day to write in your journal. Some days you won't need all ten minutes and other days you may run over. You can always find ten minutes for yourself no matter how busy you are.
- Tell others to leave you alone during your journal time. Unless the house is on fire or someone needs to go to the emergency room, nothing horrible will happen without you during those ten minutes.
- Consider writing your life story, from your earliest memories up until now. Let this take as many days or weeks as feels comfortable.
- Reflecting on your life story, identify times when you became aware of being uncomfortable or unhappy in your body. Write about those memories and what was happening in the rest of your life at that time.
- Trace the lifeline of any symptoms that arose from your eating and body obsessions. Try to identify the periods when you had the most body image difficulty, and then record the circumstances surrounding that period of your life. What might you have been hungering for at each of these points?
- Reflect on how other family members handled food, weight and body image. How did this affect you then? How does it affect you now?
- Write about what is happening in your life currently that stirs up eating or body image struggles. What is behind these struggles, and how can you support yourself better?

This short list of suggestions may keep you and your journal busy for weeks or months. From this point forward, use your journal to tune in to how you are feeling that day, identify recurring patterns in your life, and give yourself support and validation.

Notes

1 "Dear every woman I know, including me." *O, The Oprah Magazine*, November 2011. See www.oprah.com/spirit/Improving-Body-Image-How-to-Feel-Beautiful-Improving-Self-Esteem. (retrieved September 22, 2015).
2 *Appetites: Why Women Want* (Berkeley, CA: Counterpoint, 2004) p. 17.
3 Adapted from James O. Prochaska, John Norcross and Carlo DiClemente, *Changing for Good: A Revolutionary Six-Stage Program for Overcoming Bad Habits and Moving Your Life Positively Forward* (New York: William Morrow, 2007).
4 *Gracious Living in a New World: Finding Joy in Changing Times* (New York: William Morrow, 1996) p. 29.
5 Anita Johnston, *Eating in the Light of the Moon* (Carlsbad, CA: Gürze Books, 2000) p. xvii.
6 See Carolyn Costin and Joe Kelly (Eds.), *Yoga and Eating Disorders: Ancient Healing for a Modern Illness* (New York: Routledge, 2016).
7 This section on treatment models is adapted from Margo Maine, "Beyond the medical model: A feminist frame for eating disorders," In Margo Maine, William N. Davis and Jane Shure (Eds.) *Effective Clinical Practice in the Treatment of Eating Disorders: The Heart of the Matter* (London, UK: Routledge, 2009) pp. 3–17.
8 Eating Disorders Anonymous, "About EDA: Balance—not abstinence—is our goal." See www.eatingdisordersanonymous.org/about.html (retrieved August 25, 2015).
9 Craig L. Johnson and Randy A. Sansone (1993) "Integrating the twelve-step approach with traditional psychotherapy for the treatment of eating disorders." *International Journal of Eating Disorders*, 14 (2), 121–134.
10 Retrieved August 25, 2015.
11 Cited in Judith Ruskay Rabinor, *A Starving Madness: Tales of Hunger, Hope and Healing in Psychotherapy* (Carlsbad, CA: Gürze Books, 2002) p. 63.
12 Personal communication with Joe Kelly.
13 *The Happy Heretic* (Amherst, NY: Prometheus Books, 2000) p. 13.
14 *Fire in the Rain …Singer in the Storm: An Autobiography* with Derk Richardson (New York: William Morrow & Co., 1990).
15 *Coming to Our Senses: Healing Ourselves and the World Through Mindfulness* (New York: Hyperion, 2005) p. 85.
16 *Women Who Run With the Wolves* (New York: Ballantine Books, 1996) p. 364.
17 Amy Wallace, "True thighs." *More*, September, 1992. p. 92. Cited in Tim Ambler, "Questions marketers need to answer," In Jagdish N. Sheth and Rajendra S. Sisodi (Eds.) *Does Marketing Need Reform?: Fresh Perspectives on the Future* (New York: Routledge, 2006) p. 171.

9 Thinking and Coping in New Ways

In pursuit of perfection, we see every situation and phenomenon (including food and the body) as good or bad, either/or. As a result, we always feel flawed, inadequate and thwarted. We believe we're incapable of changing anything in our lives. This is because our thought patterns actually shape our reality and emotions in powerful ways. "Perfect" thinking can only create a depressing and disappointing reality.

It may seem like a dichotomous yes/no world would be safe, certain and secure. However, a dichotomous worldview is dangerously rigid, limiting and unreal. In the "perfect" illusion, we see nothing but extremes. We blind ourselves to the fact that most of real life lies in the in-between, without flawless success or unadulterated failure.

We can cope—and feel—much better if we teach ourselves to see reality's beautiful rainbow of hues between black and white. Such flexible, nuanced thinking is central to developing a positive relationship with food and our body. This means translating our feelings from the Perfect Problem's rigid language of fat into the flowing language of emotion and words. It means moving our *thoughts* away from the stifling standard of perfection and into the fresh air of imperfect reality.

> Imperfection is not our personal problem; it is a natural part of existing.[1]
>
> Tara Brach

Minding the Mind

When we think of everything as one side of a dichotomy, we virtually eliminate the ability to make progress. For example, if we believe that every situation or thought is either perfect or fatally flawed, we can't learn from our mistakes. Mistakes serve only to beat us down, rather than work as helpful lessons, teachers and opportunities to change. Black-and-white thinking convinces us that we are total losers if we *ever* slip up.

This kind of thinking is woven into eating and body image disorders. Women with these disorders judge their lives as all one way or all the

- Selective attention: We pay attention only to things that support a negative view of ourselves. We filter out facts, opinions and voices that contradict our negative view or dichotomous thinking. We hear criticisms but seem deaf to compliments.
- Oversimplification: Everything revolves around food, weight, size, appearance and shape. Nothing else about us is important.
- Superstitious thinking: We believe in cause–effect relationships where none exist. We may feel that God is punishing us through our eating disorder, that we cannot get better and that we deserve the castigation. We continue to hold these beliefs even after they are proven invalid.

Such thinking bends and twists our perception of reality. Cognitive distortion is the exaggeration of an idea, concept, or memory. The exaggeration is often over-personalized and negative—ideal for feeding eating disorders, body dissatisfaction and the quest for perfection. The solution for cognitive distortion is a technique called *cognitive restructuring*, which helps us to reframe our thoughts to reflect reality more accurately.[3]

Here's a simple exercise in cognitive restructuring to try right now. Can you hear the Voice of Perfection's negative words and thoughts in your mind? If so, write them down now.

Writing out a negative thought literally gets it out of your head, where you can examine it more coolly and subject it to critical questions like these (or others you come up with).

- Does this thought affect my behavior around food and my body? How?
- Where did I learn this thought?
- Is this thought logical?
- Is this thought actually true?
- What am I getting right now out of listening to The Voice?
- Do I want to pay that price?

Once we've written down the thought and the answers to our questions about it, the thought itself will look different because we've reexamined it in a new light. Usually, we find that the Voice of Perfection is illogical and full of falsehoods. In this simple and concrete way, we start to alter our thinking process.

The next step is to write down a *corrected* thought. We come up with a new thought based on logic, truth and reality. This cognitive restructuring process takes lots of practice before it starts to feel natural—after all, we are undoing years of old, negative, dichotomous thinking patterns. And we must remember that logic and truth alone can't magically change negative behavior or symptoms. We still have to work hard on our behavior, but now we have a new and powerful tool: our mind. Plus we can take comfort in knowing that we are starting to change one very important behavior: our thinking itself.

> Unless you feel beautiful inside, you will not see your outer beauty, let alone believe it or enjoy it. Feeling lovely is more central than looking lovely. The inner shift precedes the outer change.[4]
>
> Marcia G. Hutchinson

As we learn to correct The Voice and its destructive reasoning, we can also use a technique called *thought stopping*. When we begin to hear that negative Voice or an illogical thought, we catch ourselves and say: "Stop!" (out loud if we must), or we imagine a big red stop sign that brings the thought to a halt.

Buddhism teaches that our energy follows our thoughts. If you start to have a self-denigrating thought, no matter how distorted it is from reality, your energy suddenly follows that thought and runs away with it. We can transform our thoughts and our energy by tuning into the here and now, and by practicing a moment of non-dichotomous, non-perfectionistic thinking. This brief pause makes it easier to redirect our reasoning toward a corrected thought. We can truly change our minds and change our energy. Recovery—freeing our lives from the prison of perfectionism—requires both of those.

Finally, we can develop some quick and easy *positive retorts* to our negative thoughts. I encourage my clients to write short, simple affirmations (like "I am beautiful inside and out!"), and tape them up in prominent and problematic places around the house. Hanging in my office are mirrors that say these positive messages to my clients:

- She believes in herself
- She reaches for the stars
- In her dreams, she can fly
- Dream.

After years of hearing The Voice, cognitive distortion becomes second nature. The good news is that with daily practice, restructured, positive thinking patterns can also become second nature. When we tune in to our negative self-talk, we become more quickly aware whether cognitive distortion has kicked in, creating an opportunity to rebut The Voice and correct its distortions. Some women take a satiric approach; because they don't think The Voice deserves respect, they sass back at it. Others let loose their anger and shout back at it. No matter what our approach, we are building a real alternative to The Voice. Recovery requires developing a voice of our own and using it often.

Identifying and Correcting Negative Self-Talk

This chart gives examples of how we can take some common negative thinking from The Voice and creatively convert it into our own reality-based voice and take back control of our thinking.

Negative Self-talk (Cognitive Distortion)	Rebuttal (Cognitive Restructuring)
They all think I am fat and disgusting.	I don't know what they really think. I am not fat and disgusting. I'm just unsure of myself right now.
I always embarrass myself in social situations.	Not true. Absolute statements like "I always ..." are the kind of all-or-nothing thinking that causes me trouble. In social situations, I am actually good with other people and show a lot of caring.
Everyone is going to stare at me. I'll ruin everything if I don't look right.	They won't really care about how I look. I'm not responsible for other people, their thinking, or their feelings. Besides, no one's outward appearance has the power to determine whether or not an event is ruined.
I ate like a pig last night. Everyone will think I'm weak and out of control.	I ate a normal meal of food that my nutritionist recommended People are actually more focused on themselves, and may not even notice me.
I lost it last night. I should never have eaten that. I'll have to starve myself today.	I can't change yesterday, so I need to start over today. I don't have to punish myself for eating or for enjoying food. There are no laws against either of those.
I overheard them talking about exercise. They must think I'm fat and need to lose weight.	The world does not revolve around me. It's unlikely they were talking about me; they were probably talking about themselves.

Developing a Fuller Perception of Who We Are

> Perfectionism doesn't make you perfect. It makes you feel inadequate.[5]
> Maria Shriver

Because the pursuit of perfection and the idealization of thinness are so deeply entrenched in our culture (and in our psyches), it is easy to believe that other people care about us only for the shape our body is in. We often use that belief as a rationalization for making our body shape into the only thing we care about too. But there is a lot more to us—and to other people—than how our bodies look.

To live a healthy life, we must take time to conceptualize who we really are. This takes practice, just like cognitive restructuring does. We start with concrete steps to make ourselves conscious of our nonphysical attributes—which are far more numerous (and important) than the physical ones.

Attribute Inventory

If you write down information about your personal qualities, you literally see those traits in a new light. Write one- or two-sentence answers to the following questions. Brief answers may help you avoid convoluted rationalizations, cognitive distortions and/or other habits that denigrate your attributes. If the list of questions seems overwhelming, break it up into smaller chunks, doing two or three each day until you finish them.

- In what ways do I relate to others?
- What are my particular strengths in my relationships with my partner, friends, family, coworkers, strangers and acquaintances?
- What are my weak spots in these relationships?
- How do or would other people describe me?
- How does my view of myself fit with how other people tend to see me?
- What words best describe my personality?
- When do I feel that my very best qualities are evident? What am I likely to be doing?
- What are my values and beliefs?
- When do I feel most connected to my values and beliefs?
- In what ways do I function at work?
- What are my work habits?
- What are my strengths and weaknesses at work?
- In what ways do I handle my responsibilities at home?
- In what ways do I handle my responsibilities for self care and meeting my personal needs?
- In what ways do I handle my responsibilities for my family's needs?
- What are my intellectual strengths and weaknesses?
- What are my emotional strengths and weaknesses?
- What are my spiritual strengths and weaknesses?
- What are my hobbies, special talents and/or expertise?
- What do other people seem to like about me?

- What do I value about myself?
- What are all the things I do in a normal day? (Make a list.)
- What am I really like?
- What do I love in my life?
- What's important to me?
- What have I lost as the years have passed, but that I want to have back in my life?

Your answers to these questions can help you begin to appreciate who you really are. Each day be aware of these important personal attributes. Be aware that you are more than perfectionism says you are. Recognize that you can decide to connect your self-worth to your many rich and precious internal attributes—and disconnect your self-perception from your appearance.

Can I Get Better?

Yes, women with eating and body image disorders can get better. But eating and body image disorders are complicated in all their aspects, including the part about getting better. That means we must first talk about what we mean by *better, worse* and *recovery*. For example, women working on overcoming eating disorders often expend great effort trying to figure out if they have completely recovered. But that may not be a fruitful use of our time and energy.

On the one hand, there is no consensus regarding the criteria for recovery. Most academic research focuses on physical parameters like restoration of menstrual cycles, a certain weight-to-height ratio, or abstinence from purging—but not the quality of life. Using these limited criteria, studies find that about 40 percent of women "recover" from anorexia and bulimia. Another 35 percent see improvement, but not enough to meet the "recovery" criteria. The remaining 25 percent stay ill or die from the illnesses.[6]

In general, research on eating disorders recovery is done by experts who work with the most severely ill patients, so their numbers may not reflect the whole picture or how more typical eating disorders look. For instance, outcome research on BED and OSFED is sparse, even though those illnesses are more prevalent than anorexia and bulimia. When it comes to body image obsessions, we have very little outcome research at all. Plus the criteria for recovery from body image disorder are murky because our culture makes body dissatisfaction and obsession the norm, not the exception. All of this limits what we can learn (at least so far) from research on recovery.

On the other hand, a woman with eating disorders and body image obsessions can still get much better than she is right now, both physically and mentally—even if she has struggled with these problems for decades. These disorders include a continuum of complex difficulties and stages of progress that make it hard to nail down one single point that proves whether or not someone has reached recovery.

Perspectives on Recovery

Psychologist Beth Hartman McGilley is a leader in the field of eating disorders and has recovered herself. With this combination of personal and professional experience, she has devoted much time to thinking, talking and writing about the nature of recovery. In her perspective (and ours) recovery is more than the absence of symptoms.[7]

Being symptom-free is not the endpoint but is a beginning to a process of pro-gressing and re-gressing, moving forward and back again as you begin to reclaim your life, find your true self, and accept it with all its frailties and faults. Recovery is not about becoming perfect. Instead it is about accepting your imperfections in all their beauty.

McGilley uses the analogy of a painter who paints and then repaints a canvas. Painters frequently paint over their initial images—as if they "repented." The playwright and essayist Lillian Hellman called this pentimento, a process of "seeing and seeing again."[8] Recovery is seeing more layers to one's life, and deciding to paint new pictures over the past with a fresh appreciation of the present and future.

In practical terms, it may be more useful to think of ourselves as recover*ing*, rather than recover*ed*—recovering as an ongoing process instead of recovered as a single, relatively arbitrary, immovable standard. In pentimento parlance, that would mean we are still painting the picture of our lives, rather than finishing a portrait. Eating and body image disorders already involve a lot of measuring of ourselves against external standards that don't reflect reality very well, so we may not benefit from trying to measure recovery in exact, all-or-nothing terms. The most important thing is to work on getting healthy again.

Life itself is a continuing process, rather than an immutable point in time, so we'll make more headway if we think of recovery in similar terms. As soon as you take your first steps toward breaking the cycle of eating and body image disorders, you are on the recovery road. The bottom line:

• You have every reason to believe that you can and will get better.
• You have every reason to believe that your life will improve if you get help and refuse to give up.

Sarah experienced the entire range of eating disorder symptoms and began treatment for the first time when she was in her early forties. She was convinced that she could never make peace with her body image. It was a struggle, but she kept at it and started to see glimmers of hope.

About a year into therapy, Sarah had a transforming experience while getting ready for a holiday party. As she pulled on her panty hose, she began her usual and familiar negative self-talk of "your family is going to ridicule you behind your back because your thighs are too fat. You look terrible in this dress; no one will like you." Somehow, in the next moment, she looked in the mirror and let go of The Voice. She replaced its corrosive messages by speaking aloud: "Margo is right: I am a goddess."

I had never used those exact words with Sarah, but I had shown deep respect and unconditional positive regard for her as a person.[9] I expressed my appreciation of the many trials she had been through in her life and of her resilience and inner beauty. It was a wonderful therapeutic moment for both of us to hear her say she was starting to believe that she was a worthwhile person—in fact, a goddess.

> Belief is as necessary to the soul as pleasures are necessary to the body.[10]
>
> Elsa Schiaparelli

This was a concrete example of the new ways therapy helped Sarah to understand her life. Relational respect was teaching her that she no longer had to punish herself through her eating disorder or blame herself for family problems she did not cause. After months of hard work, soul-searching, and verbalizing things she had never shared before, Sarah found that she no longer had to translate difficult feelings into the language of fat. Instead she could deal with them directly. In turn, she could start seeing herself for who she really is. Life hasn't stopped sending challenges her way, but Sarah no longer needs to use the rituals she developed around body image and eating to cope with life's challenges. She can face them head-on instead. She no longer hides behind her attempts to craft a perfect body to "make up for" an imperfect life. And she is much happier.

Sarah's experience echoes what I have heard from clients since the 1980s, and what I learned while interviewing women in recovery for my doctoral dissertation. When I ask women in recovery what helped them to get better, the most common responses are these.

- My therapist didn't give up on me.
- I didn't feel alone anymore.

The keys to recovery—connection and hope—ring through these words. You can't do this alone. You don't have to give up. There is safety in numbers. You can get better.

> The brain is a social organ, and our relationships with one another are not a luxury but an essential nutrient for our survival.[11]
>
> Daniel Siegel

Healing Through Connection

Sarah was brave enough to give up her eating disorder, and all the related behaviors and beliefs that were her security blanket for more than 25 years. Like many others, her relationship with her eating disorder became important because of too many disappointments and injuries in significant relationships throughout her life. Eating disorder symptoms are misguided ways to soothe ourselves when we experience normal and/or extreme stressors. Growing up in a stressful and chaotic home, Sarah never learned how to calm herself, handle difficult emotions, or gain a sense of mastery or self-worth. So, she turned to the eating disorder to protect herself from further pain and which gave a false sense of control. But eating disorders did not (and do not) solve anything. While they often begin in response to deep relational disconnections, eating disorders only continue the disconnection, isolating the person from any satisfying relationships with others with their inner selves, and with their own bodies.

My approach as a therapist is to build a strong relationship which works as a bridge between the suffering person and me as a resource of concern, empathy and knowledge about eating disorders, and skills to promote recovery and wellness. The model of treatment I utilize is called Relational/Cultural Theory. RCT sees eating disorders as disorders of disconnection. The only real remedy to such disconnection is to reestablish connections with others, with one's true self, and with one's body.[12]

While traditional views of human development stress the importance of individuation and autonomy, RCT sees the importance of relationships, mutuality and empathy. Those forces were at work when Sarah saw herself in a positive light for the first time—and began to let go of her eating disorder "protection." The isolation of her eating disorder caused Sarah pain and she needed a deep interpersonal connection to disrupt the eating disorder's powerful dictates, and instill a belief that she deserved better.

New findings from the world of neuroscience reinforce the importance of relationships in the process of recovery. This research shows that the brain is basically a social organ, with mirror neurons that fire in response to the interactions we have with others. It turns out that even neuroscience shows that relationships are not luxuries; like food and water, they are essential to our survival.[13]

Relational neuroscience integrates the core principles of RCT by showing us that the human brain is "hard-wired" to connect.[14] Isolation actually causes parts of the brain to atrophy and our neural pathways to suffer. Only when we are safely connected to others does the brain get what it needs to create the neurochemistry allowing us to be calm, resilient, productive and able to function well. Our therapeutic relationship had fed Sarah's brain what it needed, so she was able to make changes in her thoughts, self-perceptions and behaviors that she never expected. The day of her insight she was doing the same thing she had done so many times: getting ready for a social event while feeling insecure and inadequate. Therapy allowed her to stop pursuing perfection for the first time, and to begin to accept herself "as is," launching her recovery process.

Neuroscience has also found that the same pain centers of the brain are activated regardless of whether the "pain" sensation comes from a physical or interpersonal source.[15] This confirms what clinicians, philosophers and theologians have always suspected: psychic or emotional pain is just as real as physical pain. Ignoring psychic pain is as foolhardy as ignoring the fact that your leg is broken.

The only road to recovery from a broken leg is to acknowledge the pain, get a doctor to identify and set the affected bone, and then follow your rehabilitation instructions (e.g., use your crutches, keep your leg elevated, don't attempt to run a marathon, etc.). We must follow the same process for the psychological pains contributing to eating disorders.

Patients frequently tell me they just want or need to "get over this." Too often people with eating disorders also get the message from others (sometimes even from their treatment providers) that they should "just eat normally." My response is that they need to get *through* it (not "over it") by uncovering the pain, experiences and beliefs that lent such power to the Voice of Perfection and to their eating and body image issues. We have to identify, understand and address these dynamics in order to reclaim our lives.

> It is in the middle of misery that so much becomes clear. The one who says nothing good comes of this is not yet listening.[16]
>
> Clarissa Pinkola Estés

Therapy starts this process—just like the X-ray and bone-setting start the process of healing a broken leg. However, most of the healing happens outside of the therapist's office (for an eating disorder) or orthopedist's office (for a broken leg). To move recovery forward, we need positive relationships outside of therapy (for eating disorders) and crutches after the X-ray (for a broken leg). In both cases, recovery is all about reconnection. Fortunately, positive relationships are far more pleasant than crutches!

Believing in Recovery

Because recovery is a long and paradoxical process, it can be hard to imagine any light at the end of the tunnel. I sometimes advise patients or their families to believe in recovery just as they once believed in Santa Claus or the tooth fairy. This is a big leap of faith—often blind faith— after years of living with the underlying conviction that you deserve the pain and misery of your eating and body image obsessions. It may seem naive or gullible to believe in recovery, but every one of us deserves to believe, just as we deserved the right to believe in Santa, and reap the rewards of that genuine trust each December.

Recovery can be a discouraging process, with a step or two forward and then a slide back. Eating disorders are powerful illnesses, much like cancers. Even with the best cancer treatment, many people do not get better in their first round of treatment. We don't blame people when they do not recover quickly from other serious illnesses, so you cannot blame yourself if recovery requires multiple stages.

> There comes a time in our lives when we are called to believe the unbelievable. If we allow ourselves to believe, we open the door to the infinite possibility of who we might become.[17]
>
> Ann Linnea

It is too daunting to attempt recovery entirely alone. An experienced therapist can help you figure out the reasons for your slips and learn from them, instead of letting them defeat you. Therapy is essential in teaching you to believe that you can have a less conflicted—or even a peaceful—relationship with food. With this guidance, experiences that once crushed you become opportunities to reshape your self-concept, worldview, beliefs and behaviors. When things look dark or you feel ambivalent, it helps to remember the 12-step saying "Don't give up five minutes before the miracle."

Louise (you read her story in Chapter 6) had every reason to give up on herself after suffering from severe bulimia for well over 20 years. She went through treatment twice, including a year-long intensive outpatient program where she made great progress. Louise and her husband devoted a lot of energy and financial resources to her recovery. But then she had a severe relapse when life events became extremely stressful.

Somehow she didn't give up. Louise decided to take a bigger step and enter residential treatment, even though it was difficult for her husband and school-age sons to have her so far away from home. Finally, this last chapter of treatment helped her to break bulimia's stubborn hold. Louise is now living fully on the recovery road, as vibrant and alive a woman as can be. Her recovery still requires attention, and she does not take it for granted, but she is grateful that she never gave up.

Life is not a Dress Rehearsal

It is normal for people to wish, from time to time, that they were younger, looked different, or were someone else. It's actually healthy to have such occasional fancies because our wishes and fantasies usually represent a deeper appetite. Say you are 55 and, one day, you are smitten with the desire to be 23 again. That wish probably springs from a longing to rekindle a warm new emotional tone in an important relationship, or resurrect the youthful freedom to explore any life direction without encumbrances.

However, it is not healthy to build your life around passing fancies or use them to define your life story. Understanding our underlying hungers keeps us from staying *stuck* in the initial fantasy or the desire to move back to an earlier time of life. If we are missing a sense of connection with our partner, we don't need a time machine that teleports us back to our first date. We need to use our experience and hope to recharge the relationship, so we can then travel forward together to new and deeper connections far more satisfying than puppy love. After all, life is a cumulative process; each day and year builds on the last. Our experience gets richer if we move forward with a willingness to learn and change. Trying to freeze time or live in the past doesn't work and brings no lasting satisfaction.

Learning how to move on is easier when we can admire the paths blazed by women before us. Some of those pioneers are people we know. Others are famous and historical women we can learn from, too (more on this in the next section).

I wasn't yet 30 when my friend Caroline turned 40. Back then, 40 seemed pretty old, but Caroline's perspective was liberating. She proudly announced: "I no longer feel compelled to buy all the back-to-college fashion magazines each August!" Her words were a great gift to me, because I saw a lively, optimistic woman embracing her age as a positive reality. I am now at an age when 40 sounds pretty *young*, but I still cherish the perspectives of my vibrant female elders. No matter how old we are, it helps to find ourselves some Carolines!

Another friend named Phoebe struggled through multiple bouts of breast cancer. Her mantra for recovery and life is: "This is not a dress rehearsal!" Her brushes with cancer put Phoebe's concerns about weight and appearance in stark perspective. She no longer cares that she can't fit into clothes she wore 30 years ago. Instead, she has a true carpe diem ("seize the day") approach to life.

When it comes to recovery and health, we need to have this same attitude. Yes, firmly entrenched bad habits can seem to have a life of their own. But we all know that putting off a decision only makes the decision harder. We can change injurious habits, and, since we are actually living and not just rehearsing, there is simply no good reason to wait.

We are deluding ourselves if we postpone work on unhealthy food and body behaviors until some elusive morning when we might wake up to find a supernatural switch that turns off our obsessions. Pie-in-the-sky epiphanies may happen in made-for-TV movies, but they seldom occur in real life. If we continue to wait for some magic moment of motivation to strike, we risk dying before we seize the opportunity to recover. Please don't wait.

Recovery from despair over eating disorders and body image requires that you have a sense of urgency about your condition. Paradoxically, recovery also requires that you give yourself permission to take the necessary time to make the difficult life changes that recovery demands. While paradoxes are often quite challenging and confusing, remember that life itself is filled with them. Paradoxes are no excuse for not living life as fully as we can. Remember the words of that wise cancer survivor: "This is not a dress rehearsal." Today may be your best chance at recovery; take that chance now, or as soon as you possibly can.

The Women We Admire

What women do you look up to? Acknowledging the value of adult women can help us feel more positive about getting older ourselves.

Make a list of the older women in your life who had an important influence on you. Then ask yourself these questions.

- What were the influences these women had on me?
- What do I value in adult women?
- Who is an example of the kind of woman I would like to be as I get older?
- How important is that woman's appearance, shape and weight to my opinion of her?
- What does "aging gracefully" mean to me?
- What could I do to honor the contributions of women?
- What can I do to emulate positive ideals rather than media images?

New Ways to Look at Women

Our culture is starving for visible role models who age gracefully and confidently. Such women exist, but they can seem invisible because they get so little attention and public praise for aging with pride.

The popularity of the movie *Something's Gotta Give* speaks to how much we want and need a different approach to women's aging. Diane Keaton won an Academy Award for her role as the mother of a young woman dating an older man (Jack Nicholson). Eventually Keaton and Nicholson become involved in a comedic romance that contrasts refreshingly to the rigid Hollywood formula of May (female)–December (male) romances.

Diane Keaton (born 1946) is also a great real-life role model for aging gracefully. Happier since giving up her self-proclaimed dependency on romantic relationships with men, she adopted two children in her fifties, and describes her life as more complete and full of love than ever. An extremely accomplished woman, Keaton began acting in comedies, then progressed to dramatic roles, and now directs and produces theatrical and television films. Meanwhile she has edited photography books, restored houses, and revels more in enjoying beauty rather than in being beautiful.[18] As Keaton wrote in her book *Let's Just Say It Wasn't Pretty*:

> I don't regret that the face I present to the world is the same I was born with. ... I hear with my ears. I eat, speak and breathe with my mouth. I have eyebrows, eyelashes and two eyes that see. That's my favorite thing about my face. I can see trees and sunsets. ... But the most thrilling aspect of my face is its ability to express feelings. All my feelings and all my emotion come out on my face—my 67-year-old face. You see, my face identifies who I am inside. It shows feelings I can't put into words. And that is a miracle, an extraordinarily ordinary miracle, one I'm not ready to change.[19]

Keaton reminds us that women need to support these realistic images, not photoshopped distortions. Actors-turned-producers like Keaton and Geena Davis have trouble finding backing for realistic films about women of all ages—what studios disparagingly call chick flicks. But we have a role to play too. If we want different images and realities for women, we must vote with our wallets. Consumer feminism could be a powerful and transforming force if we aimed it in directions like this!

Publisher Katherine Graham is another great example of someone who came into her own as a mature woman. After her husband's suicide, Graham felt totally unprepared for running the family's news media conglomerate, including the *Washington Post* and *Newsweek*—while also raising her children. But she went ahead and learned her craft. Graham's courage in backing the *Post*'s ground-breaking coverage of Watergate had an impact she never imagined beforehand.[20]

There is only one *Washington Post* to run, and we can't all win an Oscar. But Keaton and Graham (along with Maya Angelou, Mother Teresa, Alice Walker, Gloria Steinem, Condoleezza Rice, Hillary Rodham Clinton, Sandra Day O'Conner, Elizabeth Dole, Caroline Kennedy, Meryl Streep, Jamie Lee Curtis and others) show us how women can keep growing and mastering the challenges of adulthood. They are far more useful role models than any fashion model!

Women of substance help us remember what really counts: the inner self, values, beliefs, morals and the ability to love. With this insight, we may gradually see our entire female experience differently and consider letting go of our food, weight and body image obsessions.

> Sure, Fred Astaire was great, but don't forget Ginger Rogers did everything he did ... backwards and in high heels![21]
>
> Bob Thaves

Next time we are tempted to pick up a fashion magazine, let's choose a book on women's history instead. Learn more about the history of women—it will help a lot more than the latest articles about how to be sexier, skinnier and "more successful."

Granted, it is harder to find books about important women than ones about famous men (and harder to find than fashion magazines). Historically, Western culture has ignored the contributions of women. Below are a few facts about United States women. See how far this snippet of women's history can go toward clarifying what is really important about being a woman—it is not our weight or dress size!

- Women were central to indigenous life in North America.
- Women were among the first permanent European settlers in the 1600s.
- Money raised by women helped support George Washington's army.
- Women have served in every US war.
- In 1833, Prudence Crandall violated Connecticut law by opening the first school for African-American girls.
- In 1850, Harriet Tubman escaped slavery and then returned to free 300 other slaves.
- In 1852, Harriet Beecher Stowe wrote the wildly popular and controversial abolitionist classic *Uncle Tom's Cabin*.
- Victoria Woodhull was the first woman to run for president—in 1872.
- A hundred years later, at age 47, Shirley Chisholm became the first African-American woman to run for president.
- Laura Ingalls Wilder' published her first book, *Little House in the Big Woods*, when she was 65.
- The renowned painter Anna Mary Robertson Moses (better known as Grandma Moses) started her 25-year career at age 76, when her hands were too crippled by arthritis to hold an embroidery needle.
- Julia Child didn't begin her long-running PBS program *The French Chef* until she was 51.
- Former Milwaukee public school teacher Golda Meir became Israel's first female prime minister at age 70.
- Women invented (among many other things): submarine lamps, suspenders, windshield wipers, life rafts, fire escapes, paper bags, the original Monopoly® game, the circular saw, Scotchguard®, Kevlar®, signal flares, the dishwasher and the retractable dog leash.

Entire social movements have been started by women, including these:

- In 1843, Dorothea Dix exposed abuse of the mentally ill in hospitals and paved the way for more humane treatment of psychiatric patients.
- Clara Barton founded the Red Cross in 1881.
- After decades of advocating for miners, textile workers and children, Mary Harris Jones, nicknamed "Mother Jones," led a 125-mile march of child workers to bring the evils of child labor to the attention of the President and the national press in 1903.
- In 1924, women founded the Parent–Teacher Association
- Jane Addams won the Nobel Peace Prize in 1931 for promoting mediation during World War I and for her leadership of the Women's International League for Peace and Freedom.
- Frances Perkins became the first woman member of a US cabinet in 1933. As Secretary of Labor, she was instrumental in establishing unemployment benefits, the 40-hour work week and the first minimum wage.
- In the early 20th century, Alice Hamilton was the first physician to study occupational diseases, leading to today's Workers' Compensation laws.
- In 1962, Rachel Carson's writings stimulated development of the environmental movement.
- After being forced to retire at 65, Maggie Kuhn founded the Gray Panthers in 1970 to challenge discrimination against older people.
- As a child (and with her father's encouragement), Malala Yousafzai began blogging and advocating for girls to be educated in her native Pakistan. At 15, she was shot and severely injured in an assassination attempt while boarding her school bus. At 17, Malala became the youngest-ever Nobel Peace Prize winner.

This is a tiny sampling of what women have done (and still do) to enhance the shape we're in as a society. However, contemporary culture's pursuit of perfectionism tends to keep these contributions hidden. That is why women's history is so useful in changing how we see ourselves. When we replace the narrow cultural view of women with a new appreciation of our many historic accomplishments, we start changing the standards by which we judge our own success and value.

In becoming archaeologists of the world of our mothers, we are trying to retrieve the female past and to invent a future.[22]

Louise Bernikow

Scanning the Past

Our own family history can go a long way in helping us live healthfully and in recovery. Look over old family photos, portraits, or videos to learn what the bodies in our family are supposed to be like and what our genetic heritage means for our sense of self. This historical research is instructive while also being a lot of fun!

As you look at images of your ancestors, consider these questions.

- What are the women's body types like?
- What relative do you most resemble in body type or appearance?
- What stories of female accomplishment can you see or remember when you look at the images?
- What do the women's bodies say to you?
- What relative do you most resemble in personal characteristics and accomplishment?
- What do your relatives and their stories teach you about being female?
- What do they teach you about attractiveness?
- What do they teach you about getting older?
- What do they teach you about sexuality?
- What do you feel about these people?
- What do you feel about their bodies?
- What do you feel about your own body as you look at theirs?

We have a lineage and legacy of accomplishment, body shape and true beauty. Seeing photos of relatives we love or admire can help us to love and admire the parts of us they passed down to us. Images in the family photo album can offer a far better reflection of reality than magazines or TV shows. Appreciate the bodies, beauty and accomplishments of our female ancestors. That can do a lot to help us appreciate ourselves.

Notes

1 *Radical Acceptance: Embracing Your Life with the Heart of a Buddha* (New York: Bantam, 2004) p. 21.
2 *Eat, Pray, Love* (New York: Riverhead Books, 2007) p. 57.
3 Alice D. Domar and Henry Dreher, *Self-Nurture: Learning to Care for Yourself As Effectively As You Care for Everyone Else* (New York: Penguin Books, 2001).
4 Marcia G. Hutchinson, *Transforming Body Image: Learning to Love the Body You Have* (Berkeley, CA: The Crossing Press, 1985) p. 14.

5 *Ten Things I Wish I'd Known – Before I Went Out into the Real World* (New York: Grand Central, 2000) p. 61.

6 American Psychiatric Association (2000) "Practice guidelines for the treatment of patients with eating disorders (revision)." *American Journal of Psychiatry*, 157 (1), 1–39.

7 Beth Hartman McGilley and Jacqueline K. Szablewski (2010) "Recipe for recovery: Necessary ingredients for the client's and clinician's success," In Margo Maine, Beth Hartman McGilley and Douglas Bunnell (Eds.) *Treatment of Eating Disorders: Bridging the Research–Practice Gap.* (London: Elsevier, 2010) p. 23.

8 *Pentimento* (Boston, MA: Little, Brown and Company, 1973) p. 3.

9 See Carl Rogers, *On Becoming a Person: A Psychotherapists View of Psychotherapy* (Boston, MA: Mariner Books, 1995).

10 *Shocking Life: The Autobiography of Elsa Schiaparelli* (New York: E. P. Dutton, 1954) p. 23.

11 *Mindsight: The New Science of Personal Transformation* (New York: Bantam, 2010) p. 211.

12 Karen L. Samuels and Margo Maine (2012). "Treating eating disorders at midlife and beyond: Help, hope, and the Relational Cultural Theory." *Work in Progress: No. 110.* Jean Baker Miller Training Institute at Wellesley Centers for Women.

13 Daniel J Siegel, *Mindsight: The New Science of Personal Transformation* (New York: Bantam Books, 2011).

14 Amy Banks and Leigh Ann Hirschman, *Four Ways to Click: Rewire Your Brain for Stronger, More Rewarding Relationships* (Crows Nest, New South Wales: Allen & Unwin, 2015).

15 Naomi I. Eisenberger and Matthew D. Lieberman (2004) "Why rejection hurts: A Common neural alarm system for physical and social pain." *Trends in Cognitive Science*, 8 (7), 294–300.

16 *Women Who Run With the Wolves* (New York: Ballantine, 1996) p. 384.

17 *Deep Water Passage: A Spiritual Journey at Midlife* (New York: Little, Brown and Company, 1995) p. 186.

18 Margot Dougherty, "Diane Keaton: The art of being yourself." *More*, May 2014. See www.more.com/entertainment/celebrities-movies-tv-music/diane-keaton-more-magazine-may-2014-the-art-of-being-yourself (retrieved August 24, 2015).

19 New York: Random House, 2014, p.29.

20 *Personal History* (New York: Vintage Books, 1998).

21 See Rosalie Maggio, *The New Beacon Book of Quotations by Women* (Boston, MA: Beacon Press, 1996) p. 451: "Widely quoted and most often attributed to [the late Texas Governor] Ann Richards, although she always disclaimed authorship, this remark apparently first appeared in a comic strip by Bob Thaves. In *Ginger: My Story* (New York: HarperCollins, 1991) p. 137, Ginger Rogers writes: 'A friend sent me a cartoon called "Frank and Ernest" from an LA newspaper. It showed Fred on a sandwich board announcing a "Fred Astaire Festival." A woman was standing near the sandwich board, talking to Frank and Ernest. The balloon coming out of her mouth said, "Sure, he was great, but don't forget that Ginger Rogers did everything he did … backwards and in high heels!"' The cartoon was copyright 1982.'

22 *Among Women* (New York: HarperCollins, 1981) p. 46.

10 Embracing Our Selves

The perfection that humanity seeks can only be found in the present moment, and nowhere else.[1]

Arran Anderson

Life is not a destination but a journey of self-discovery and self-nurturance, best lived when we are intentionally doing things to stay well and to improve our emotional and spiritual state. It is never too late to accept our imperfections and start this journey. Whether we're 30 or 80, we can decide to dump the pursuit of perfection (and its either/or lens of evaluating success/failure), reclaim our life, focus on our own values and desires, and embrace our shape and self.

The Legacy We Leave

Many factors help us get beyond perfectionism and keep a healthy body image—starting with the values and core beliefs that guide us. These life fundamentals are best revealed in the fundamental questions we ask ourselves each day. At war with our bodies and confused about our true hungers and needs, do we use the quick fix of our appearance to measure our personal value and our public success? How much energy do we expend cross-examining our bodies and other women's bodies? Does looking for answers in unattainable perfection leave us empty and hungering for more?

Far too many of us ask more questions about the shape our bodies than the shape of our emotional, relational and spiritual lives.

We must abandon the pressure to be perfect, and replace it with fundamental questions like "Who do I want to be?" and "What do I want?"

Our perspective changes for the better when our questions move away from the mirror and the compulsion to please other people through our appearance. Then we can focus on contributing to the world and pleasing ourselves through our core being. Only then can we embrace our beautifully imperfect selves and lives, pursue happiness, and live fully.

So what *is* it that makes us happy, keeps us happy, and gives life meaning?

- A trip to the mall, or a walk with a friend?
- A talk with your partner, or a couple of hours at the gym?
- Weighing a pound less, or nurturing deep connections with others?

Many of us are much better at preparing to live a "perfect" life than to actually live our own life. Pursuing perfection is not our only option. Instead of waiting until we get "the right stuff" (or the right body), we can start living more fully with what we have, and in our deliciously imperfect bodies, right now. This *real* stuff will displace the power that dissatisfaction with appearance (including eating disorders and body image despair) hold in our lives. Then we will be able to embrace our real body and live more richly.

Life's fundamental questions are actually pretty simple, but they are not easy—especially in today's culture. We have to find ways to avoid being distracted by "the right stuff" and discover "the real stuff" that is important to us.

A famous conversation in the Margery Williams children's classic *The Velveteen Rabbit* clarifies a fundamental life purpose: becoming real and being loved.

> "What is REAL?" asked the Rabbit one day ... "Does it mean having things that buzz inside you and a stick-out handle?"
>
> "Real isn't how you're made," said the Skin Horse. "It's a thing that happens to you. When a child really loves you for a long, long time, not just to play with, but REALLY loves you, then you become Real ... It doesn't happen all at once ... You become. It takes a long time ... Generally, by the time you are Real, most of your hair has been loved off, and your eyes drop out and you get loose in the joints and very shabby. But these things don't matter at all, because once you are Real you can't be ugly, except to people who don't understand."[2]

One simple (but not easy) way to decide what's important in life is to consider the epitaph we want on our tombstone, or what we hope our obituary will say. Do we want to be remembered as "a good dieter," or as "a great friend?" Do we want "she slimmed down to a size 6," or "she used her boundless energy to make the world a better place"? Do we want our dearest friends to think of us as coldly perfectionistic, or as warmly quirky and loveable?

> Vulnerability is not weakness. It fuels our daily lives. Vulnerability is our most accurate measurement of courage.[3]
>
> Brené Brown

Today it is easy to feel inconsequential as our busy world races by, filled with the pursuit of perfection, fame and celebrity. But we are not perfect—*or* inconsequential. We affect people, especially the ones we love, in big ways and small. (If you think little things don't matter, remember your last mosquito bite.)

We need to decide what mark we want to leave on this earth and on the people we touch. How do we want to be remembered? Let's imagine our future legacy and strive to create a life that lives up to it.

A Moment's Peace

We are the first generation with smart phones, smart watches, texting, email, tablets, laptops and other telecommunications miracles. We are plugged-in pioneers, expected to manage all kinds of input and stressors we couldn't imagine even ten years ago.

As contemporary women, we have come to accept electronic interruption as normal. People can access us instantly to get anything from us. Always on call, we often feel pressured to provide a perfect response.

> When I think about, say, 1995, or whenever the last moment was before most of us were on the internet and had mobile phones, it seems like a hundred years ago. ... Time passed in fairly large units, or at least not in milliseconds and constant updates. A few hours wasn't such a long time to go between moments of contact with your work, your people, or your trivia.[4]
>
> Rebecca Solnit

Access to 24/7 international news is also stressful; we deal with our day-to-day responsibilities while also witnessing what is happening all over the globe. Tragic and frightening news seeps into our consciousness and often creates vicarious trauma. Living in a state of hyper-arousal, the smallest and most mundane issues may take on undue significance and urgency, leaving us to feel overwhelmed much of the time.

There are advantages to all this sophisticated technology. But moments of calm, peace, or reflection are rare, even though these moments are essential for our well-being and healthy development. Constant distractions cloud our inner feelings and wisdom—keeping us from knowing our true hungers. Some of us actually keep ourselves hooked into all those electronics specifically to avoid ourselves and how we really feel.

We have to find ways to create quiet time for reflection in our life. In fact, former patients sometimes tell me that being able to "sit by myself and do nothing" is an essential ingredient in recovery. We need to find moments of peace and quiet on a regular basis to embrace ourselves and reclaim our lives.

Mindfulness

How often do we pay attention to ourselves and our world fully, purposefully and without judgment? Mindfulness is a practice that makes us more aware, in tune and in touch with each moment. Many spiritual practices (including Buddhism, Taoism, Christianity, yoga, indigenous spiritualities and transcendentalism) hold mindfulness as central to spiritual growth. When we practice being in touch and at one with our inner world and senses, we begin to awaken to our own true nature.

Although mindfulness is part of formal meditation practices, it is also a very simple method of awareness. Buddhist thinking describes mindfulness as "Beginner's Mind," a fresh way of looking at the world with eyes wide open to notice and appreciate what is within and around us. Mindfulness increases our ability to see the miracles and beauty in our imperfect world, like the sky, the wind, trees—and our miraculous bodies. Mindfulness also helps redirect us from the distractions of modern life to become more spiritual and appreciative of important intangibles, like love.

Paradoxically, mindfulness means *thinking* a little less and *sensing* a little more. As we increase our awareness of the phenomena that our five senses experience, we begin to unite the body and the mind. Rather than keeping our mind and body at war with each other, mindfulness can help us to understand that we are human "beings." Too often we see ourselves as human "doings," only worthwhile for our accomplishments. But a human being's true value stems more from who she is than for what she does.

Mindful Breathing

Most of the time, our bodies are doing one thing and our minds are thinking about something else. Through mindful breathing, the two can come together.[5] Here's a simple technique to begin this process. Sit or lie quietly, and then:

- Breathe in slowly, deeply, and say to yourself "in."
- Breathe out slowly and say to yourself "out."
- After doing this for a few minutes you will feel calmer and clearer, more mindful.
- Or, upon breathing in, say, "Breathing in, I calm my body."
- And upon breathing out, say, "Breathing out, I smile."

Mindfulness helps us choose our responses to life situations, rather than mind*less*ly reacting. Since we are more aware of the circumstances and what we feel, emotions don't have to ambush or overwhelm us. We choose to react consciously, rather than reflexively.

Mindfulness also enables us to focus on the present, instead of rehashing the past (the food we should not have eaten) or worrying about the future (the pounds we will lose or gain). In the end, happiness is really only possible in the present, because we can't change the past or control the future. Thus, through our mindfulness, we help to create happiness.

Time was a river, not a log to be sawed into lengths.[6]

Margaret A. Robinson

We actually design our own reality in many ways. For example, if you choose to smile, you relax hundreds of muscles throughout your entire body. According to Buddhist teacher Thich Nhat Hahn, smiling is "mouth yoga" because it calms our nervous systems and instantly changes our experience.[7]

The next time we look in the mirror, let's remember to stay in the present, not berate ourselves for what we did to our body in the past, or plan future attacks on it. Smile genuinely and accept your smile back in return.

We take care of the future best by taking care of the present now.[8]

Jon Kabat-Zinn

Balance

Modern women live hectic and overloaded lives with long lists of "have-tos" and "shoulds." The pressure to be perfect's list of "shoulds" seems infinite. Trying to do it all perfectly produces exhaustion and burnout, making it easier to revert to the soothing and numbing rituals of disordered eating and body image distress. There's no better setup for emotional, physical and spiritual crisis than being exhausted and spent.

"Shoulding" all over ourselves actually strengthens our belief that—left to our own devices—we cannot be trusted. Because so much of our behavior is driven by "should," we are losing our ability to distinguish what we really "want."

Even if your actions remain unchanged, simply identifying your choice as a "should" or "want" is meaningful, and will help you know your true motivations and intentions, and thus—know yourself.[9]

Nancy Colier

If we "should" all over ourselves, we throw our entire life out of balance. Creating balance starts with basic self-care. No cosmetic product for creating a youthful appearance or household appliance for a perfect home can perform this task. Instead, the pursuit of perfection prevents us from truly taking care of ourselves. Rest and relaxation have to be part of our daily self-talk and schedule, not just something we encourage others to do, or only do ourselves during a rare vacation. Many of us "talk the talk" of self-nurturance without "walking the walk."

It may sound impossible to build relaxation time into our days, but it isn't. We simply need to reject all-or-nothing formulas of needing to do everything perfectly, including relaxation and recovery. Some days leave little time for us, but we can usually capture a few minutes to do one healthy, soothing thing for our souls. It can be as easy as having a second cup of coffee, reading a book leisurely, or another simple indulgence that helps us rest, rejuvenate and relax.

The Three Rs: Rest, Rejuvenate, Relax

Here are rest, relaxation and rejuvenation activities most of us can do without taking too much time or trouble. Add some of your own.

- Buy a coloring book and crayons, and then color like you did when you were a kid.
- Listen to your favorite music. Let yourself feel the rhythm. Dance!
- Go for a walk outdoors.
- If you can't leave home, take an imaginary walk in one of your favorite outdoor scenes.
- Call a friend or family member that you enjoy talking to.
- Read poetry—or write some.
- Take a nap.
- Watch your favorite TV show.
- Buy flowers for yourself. Admire their beauty and yours.
- Have a cup of tea or other soothing, warm drink—but not too much caffeine!
- Play solitaire.
- See a play, a movie, or a concert.
- Visit a museum or read a book about a favorite artist.
- Pray.
- Sing some old favorite songs with no one listening.
- Meditate.
- Stretch.
- Swing on a swing set.
- Watch children play at a playground.
- Beat a drum.
- Indulge in a warm bubble bath.
- Burn a candle in one of your favorite scents. Stare at the flame and relax.
- Daydream.

- Watch the sun come up or go down.
- Star gaze.
- Spend time outside. Let Mother Nature awe you.
- Listen to the birds.
- Read for pleasure.
- Plan or plant a garden.
- Spend time with a favorite pet or go to the humane society and pet a lonely animal.
- Go to a park or nature preserve.
- Return to an old hobby that you enjoy.
- Make a list of hobbies that you have wanted to pursue, and then try one.
- Browse through a library or bookstore.
- Make a collage.
- Write in your journal.
- Make a list of your favorite people. Remember a fun or special moment with each of them.
- Look at photos of family, friends, or a happy memory. Soak up that energy.
- Smile.

The Essentials

Sleep deprivation and being overtired confuse our internal body systems. Perplexed about its states and needs, the body may signal that we're hungry when we really need sleep, or suggest napping when we really need food. The only way to avoid this confusion is to be sure we are getting adequate rest and food. In fact, the healthiest older people have very steady habits of eating and sleeping[10]. Our bodies seem to handle essential life-giving processes and external stressors better when we give them balance and routine, rather than chaos or irregularity.

> "I don't have time" is the single most frequently given reason for living fractional, perpetually indentured lives, for not living fully or freely. Because time is life, when we say we don't have enough time, we are admitting that we don't have enough life.[11]
>
> Sonia Johnson

Routine sleep patterns are especially important in maintaining recovery. Going to bed and getting up at similar (but not rigidly enforced) times helps our bodies to get into a rhythm more conducive to sleep—and emotional health. Turning the world off at a reasonable hour is difficult to accomplish these days, but still essential. Let voice mail earn its keep and tell friends or colleagues how late we will accept calls and texts. Turn off the Facebook, Instagram and Twitter notifications; if something is truly an emergency, people will find us the way they did before cell phones.

It also helps to end our household tasks at a reasonable hour. Even if we have children at home, we can make some quiet time after they are in bed to do nothing, or to do something genuinely enjoyable. Keep chores in perspective—our children will remember and value us for who we are, not our housework. We need to rest even during menopause's sleep-disrupting hot flashes and night sweats, or during other emotionally straining times when sleep is elusive. If we wake up early and can't get back to sleep, enjoy those hours to relax in bed before the day starts, or use the breathing and relaxation exercises described in this chapter.

Priorities, Priorities, Priorities

We tend to live in a state of urgency about the many daily demands and opportunities of life, but very few of them are really life-and-death. Stop and think about where you were one year ago today. Can you remember specifically and in detail the biggest worry you had that day? Most of us can't, because most days don't bring memorable, earth-shattering crises. Keep that in mind when responding to *today's* worries.

Creating priorities means setting limits. Many of us agonize over choosing—and especially saying no. I tell my patients, "No is the new Yes," because mindfully establishing priorities and limits is a major step toward living well and preventing relapse into disordered symptoms. In fact, developing the ability to say no is a form of self-nurturance.

For example, most of us work both inside and outside of our homes. Yet, many of us still that feel our house must constantly look perfect, lest it (and us) be judged poorly by others. Meanwhile, research consistently shows that women carry far more of the load around home than men do, even in dual working couples. Beyond that, the presence of a husband creates disproportionately more housework for a household.

According to University of Michigan economist Frank Stafford, longitudinal research of 8,000 US families shows that:

> Single women with no children did a little more than 10 hours of housework a week [in 2005], and married women with no children did a little more than 17 hours a week. The only difference? The presence of a husband, which costs women seven hours of housework a week.
>
> For men, the situation is reversed. Single men with no children did about eight hours of housework a week, while married men with no children did a bit more than seven hours of housework a week. So a wife saves them about an hour of work a week.[12]

That makes housework feel like an endless priority, especially on a sunny day when you can see the cobwebs. A healthy, balanced life usually requires reducing the futile compulsion for a dust-free domicile. When we lessen our "perfect home" priority, we soon see that going out into the sunshine will not end the world or make the house uninhabitable.

Another simple limit-setting tactic is making a list with our partner or roommate, agreeing about what needs to be done around the house over the next two weeks. When we negotiate "chore frequency," we:

- Gain perspective on the importance of a task to the running of our home
- Gain perspective on the importance of a task to our spouse or partner, who we may think (mistakenly, perhaps) "needs" us to be compulsive about chores
- Establish a shared priority list
- Make it much easier to share the responsibility equally
- Free up new time we can take regularly for ourselves.

Too often we make housework a way to avoid other more important issues. We can't know what we really want when we keep ourselves in constant motion accomplishing inconsequential missions. We don't have to live in a hyper-alert state in our homes. Our physical appearance isn't as important as what goes on inside us—it isn't even close. The same holds true for our home—it is what happens inside that counts, not how it looks.

Learning to Breathe

Watch a baby breathe. Her belly goes visibly up and down, naturally feeding her brain adequate oxygen. All of us are born knowing how to breathe fully. Over the years, we lose this natural ability as shallow breathing becomes the norm, especially for women.

By preadolescence we're taught to "hold your stomach in," constantly contracting our abdominals in preparation for a lifetime of body consciousness and self-criticism. When we don't reclaim our right to breathe deeply and abundantly, we don't get adequate oxygen to our brains. This causes a chain reaction: without sufficient oxygen, we can't relax and our anxiety increases. In fact, most of us don't consciously recognize the change—after years of holding our stomachs in, anxiety and shallow breathing seem second nature to us.

It helps to understand the physiology of breathing. When we inhale, oxygen crosses the lung's membranes, and enters our bloodstream. Our red blood cells, rich with oxygen, engage in intracellular respiration. Our cells use the oxygen to grow, repair and replicate. Exhaling keeps us safe by removing carbon dioxide. The quality of our breathing affects *every* process in our bodies.

We'll feel better both physically and emotionally if we learn to breathe more fully. Even a short period of deep, slow breathing can lower blood pressure and reduce our anxiety level. Taking ten deep breaths before we react to a demanding or irritating situation will increase our level of calm and perspective. When we are nervous, slowing down our breathing helps us speak clearly and truly. We can do this anywhere and anytime to improve the quality of our lives. If we still struggle with anxiety about eating, using one of the breathing techniques described below before meals may help.

Breathing better and more fully feels good, once we learn how to retrain our bodies. We can also practice deep breathing in preparation for stressful times.

Belly breathing—reengaging our diaphragms rather than keeping the stomach sucked in—takes practice. Once we retrain our bodies to breathe deeply, we will benefit emotionally, physically and spiritually. Learn from the wisdom of babies.

Better Breathing Made Easy[13]

Deep Breathing

Lie on your back with your palms up and legs relaxed (the corpse pose in yoga). Consciously release the tension in all of your muscles. Slowly inhale, wait a beat, and then slowly exhale. Pay attention to the sound of your breath. Notice your belly rising and falling with each breath. Repeat for five minutes the first time around. Gradually extend the time period whenever you do the exercise. You also can do this sitting in a chair, cross-legged on the floor, or by putting your forehead down on a table, if that feels safer.

Three-Part Breathing

Sit in a chair or on the floor, with your spine straight. Inhale by expanding the abdomen. Move the breath up to the rib cage and then into the upper chest. Exhale doing the reverse, beginning at the collarbone and emptying the breath down to the stomach. Try to expel all the carbon monoxide, contracting your lower abdominal muscles to push the air out. Let your breath rise and fall, placing your fingertips on your torso to help guide the breath. Begin with one minute, then increase to four to five minutes.

Do not try to do these exercises perfectly.

Don't judge how well you are following the directions or compare yourself to someone else. The goal is to practice *relaxed* breathing so that you can do it easily and discreetly for yourself. Try to practice one of these techniques each day.

Building Breathing Room

Learning to breathe fully is one thing, but creating more breathing room in our lives is another. Both are essential to getting and staying well.

Some people around us may seem (or be) disappointed when we set limits and reclaim more of our life and energy. But none of us can be all things to all people. True friends and loved ones will respect our self-care, especially if we explain our recovery journey and the reasons we are making changes. As difficult as it may be, staying consistent with these limits will actually help others to accept and respect the breathing room we are working to establish. Not only that, but clearer boundaries actually help us establish greater connection and intimacy with the people around us! (One of life's wonderful paradoxes.)

Most of us grew up learning to acquiesce to other people's needs, leaving our own to the side. Nevertheless, we have the right to say yes and/or no to the demands in our lives. There may even be rights in our life and our relationships that we have not exercised yet.

Exercise Your Own Bill of Rights

Pick some of the rights listed here, add some of your own, and personalize your own Bill of Rights. Review your rights periodically and be sure that your life reflects them; if it doesn't, make some changes.

I have the right to:

- Speak my mind
- Ask for what I need
- Ask for what I want
- Change my mind
- Make my own decisions
- Have my own values, beliefs and priorities
- Experience a whole range of feelings
- Express my feelings, even if others won't like it
- Be honest
- Expect honesty from others
- Be angry
- Make mistakes
- Be imperfect
- Be responsible for my behavior and no one else's
- Set limits
- Say no when others ask for or expect things that interfere with meeting my own needs at that time
- Feel safe in my relationships
- Feel respected by others

- Be healthy
- Be in charge of my own life
- Pursue happiness
- Pursue my own dreams and desires
- Change and grow
- Live my life to the fullest
- Feel good in my body and about my body.

In order to say yes fully to life, women have to be able to say no.

Setting the boundary of "no" is an ongoing theme in the treatment and recovery process for women with eating and body image issues. That's because we lose track of our own basic needs for food and self-nurturance when we respond to others' needs before our own.

My father frequently said, "If you are strong enough to act on your beliefs, then not pleasing other people is just part of life." He would also paraphrase a famous quote attributed to Abraham Lincoln[14] and say, "You can please all the people some of the time, and some of the people all the time, but you cannot please all the people all the time."

Although my dad usually made these statements in conversations about public or political stands, I gradually applied the message to my internal and interpersonal life. It continues to help me balance the pressure between pleasing others and pleasing myself. My dad was right: we simply can't please all the people all the time, even if we are taught that we should. Take that great gift from my dad and keep it in your heart too.

A New Relationship with Food

If we are suffering from eating or body image disorders—or only indoctrinated with the myth of perfection—we need an entirely different relationship to our body and food in order to be healthy again. We have to learn how to see our food and our body as two necessary and wonderful givens.

If we are women who have gone without food for long periods of time, we may think we have proven that we don't need or want it. But thinking doesn't make it so.

We do need to eat. We do need to accept our imperfect bodies for what they are.

Many adult women in recovery continue to struggle with their feelings about food, and have strong desires to restrict, binge and/or purge. Nevertheless, they do learn ways to manage those emotions and make a daily commitment to eat and to take care of themselves.

It can and does work. Both Beth and her mother struggled with eating disorders for decades. But after hard work and commitment to getting better, Beth is self-regulating her feelings about food, rather than having them control her:

> Now I eat because it's the right thing to do. Not because I want to—I don't. But I know it's the right thing to do. For me. For my daughters. It's still hard and sometimes I absolutely hate food. Maybe I always will. But I eat because it's right.

Some women recovering from eating disorders tend to become overly rigid about food intake, creating complex rules because they feel a need to eat perfectly at all times. This strategy may help very early in the recovery process, but as time passes, rigidity backfires. If we don't develop food flexibility, we will still feel remorse and guilt when we give in to cravings or eat more than our bodies can handle easily because it tastes so good. That easily restarts a cycle of backsliding into symptoms, and renewed negative feelings.

When we let go of perfectionistic inflexibility, we discover that our rigid rules weren't really about the food after all. Instead they manifested:

- the deprivation we impose on ourselves in the pursuit of perfection
- our discomfort with our natural desires
- complicated emotions that food, weight and eating have masked for so long.

Most of my patients are frightened when I suggest that they loosen up the rules and allow "forbidden" foods back into their lives. It can take a long time to become convinced that there's no such thing as good food or bad food.

Dichotomous thinking about food is actually dangerous. Even eating "too much of a good thing" by excluding everything except vegetables or fruits may lead to orthorexia's severe medical problems: lost muscle stores, exhausted immune system, unsafe blood chemistries, gastrointestinal problems and a weakened heart.

Healthy living and eating include an overall balance in our nutritional intake. Unless we have specific medical reasons (such as diabetes, prescription drug interactions, or a food allergy), we can incorporate all kinds of food in our diets—and still be healthy. If most of our food choices are healthy, it is fine to incorporate some richer or less nutritious foods. Getting adequate calories and an adequate balance of fat, carbs and protein will make us less likely to overdo less healthy choices.

The human body has been functioning in balance for millennia. We have to:

- trust the innate knowledge of our long genetic history
- trust our bodies to use up what they take in

- trust that our appetites will normalize once we loosen up our rules a bit
- trust that our relationship to food will improve.

Instead of trying to be perfect (an impossibility), we need to set flexible goals, such as choosing to make 80 to 90 percent of our food choices "healthy" and use the balance to welcome in some "forbidden" foods. Despite the initial apprehension, many women feel more satisfaction and fewer cravings after increasing their flexibility in food thinking and food habits. This is a change we can live with, unlike the impossible script of perfect eating that can literally kill us.

A Different Approach to Weight and Health

So, is it possible to assess our lives and our health by standards other than our weight, size and appearance? Yes, although it's often hard to see how while besieged by our culture's relentless—and frequently misguided— "War on Obesity."

When we conflate weight with health, we ignore decades of science while creating more problems than we solve. To take one relevant example, weight stigma leads many people into perpetual cycles of dieting that disrupt health—and bring no permanent weight loss. Chronic dieting can result in a full range of clinical eating disorders from severe restricting and weight loss, to purging through exercise, laxatives, vomiting or other means, and to binge eating disorder. Despite their desire to meet the thin ideal, most dieters actually gain weight due to the ways that restrictive dieting disrupts metabolic function and the likelihood of rebound binges after extreme deprivation.

We are each unique. Therefore, reducing "health" to a number on a scale or chart is not very useful—and can be dangerous.[15] Science repeatedly demonstrates that we can be fit and "fat," or "thin" and very out of shape. Our health habits and histories—not our weight or BMI— determine our well-being.[16]

My patients and I often turn to the Health At Every Size (HAES) movement because it articulates a sane and balanced alternative to the widespread, weight-obsessed approaches in our mainstream medical system. HAES emphasizes the need to base nutritional and behavioral recommendations on the individual person's medical presentation and history—including risk patterns, genetic predispositions and other factors. Its basic principles are:

- Respect for all bodies, regardless of shape, weight, or appearance.
- Compassionate care and self-care, including non-judgmental acceptance of diverse bodies and their needs.
- Promoting attuned movement, eating habits and other self-care behaviors.

Essentially, HAES (and many scientists) argue that the keys to health are consistent and balanced nutritional intake with a full complement of foods and healthy activity levels.

At first glance, this perspective seems radical or bizarre because it has nothing to do with calories, weight, or BMI. Instead, HAES maintains a critical eye toward cultural and medical assumptions about weight, asserting that the war on obesity is based on erroneous interpretations of selected research about weight and size. HAES urges that much greater attention be given to more comprehensive research which suggests that our health depends on factors far more complicated than weight.[17]

> The scale can only give you a numerical reflection of your relationship with gravity.[18]
>
> Steve Maraboli

Unfortunately, many approaches to obesity prevention in the US ignore social determinants of health, including wide-accepted forms of prejudice based toward people with large body sizes.[19] Weight stereotypes assume that "fat" people are lazy, gluttonous and lack the willpower to practice self-discipline. Because these characteristics undermine the pursuit of perfection, we tend to disdain people we perceive as "fat," and feel justified discriminating against them in social situations—and even in the workplace.[20]

We seldom acknowledge how weightism creates adversity for people of size. Weight bias contributes to higher health risks, including depression and anxiety, negative self-image, suicidal thoughts and unhealthy attempts to lose weight. Large people are also more likely to avoid health care services due to the prejudice and negative interactions they often encounter in a system overly focused on weight and BMI. The impact on large women's health and well-being is especially significant.[21]

We also tend to ignore the relationship between profit incentives and the weight-centered paradigm of health. In fact, people in the US spent $60.5 *billion* on weight loss goods and services in 2013.[22] The global weight loss industry is growing by nearly 11 percent per year with 2014 income projected at $586.3 billion.[23] With so much money at stake, dieting and pharmaceutical companies have considerable incentives to create desperate customers fearful of the health implications of "un-lost" weight.

It is time for a radical—and realistic—shift in our attitudes and outlook toward health and weight concerns. A more comprehensive perspective focused on individual needs will get us more in tune with our own bodies, bring us closer to health—and eliminate the need to stigmatize people who don't "meet" arbitrary standards like BMI.

Our well-being depends on ending the Body Wars and trading in the pursuit of perfection for body peace.

25 Ways to Love Your Body[24]

Making peace with our bodies takes practice. Spend at least five minutes a day reflecting on this list alone, with your partner, or with family and friends. Share your reactions and experiences as you ponder the amazing things our bodies do.

1. We are born in love with our bodies. Watch an infant sucking her fingers and toes, with no awareness of or worry about body fat. Imagine being in love with your body.
2. Think of your body as a tool. Make an inventory of all the things you can do with it.
3. Notice what your body does each day. It is the instrument of your life, not an ornament for someone else's enjoyment.
4. Create a list of people you admire who have contributed to your life, your community, or the world. Was their appearance important to their accomplishments?
5. Consider your body as a source of pleasure. Think of all the ways it can make you feel good.
6. Enjoy your body: stretch, dance, walk, sing, take a bubble bath, get a massage, or get a pedicure.
7. Put signs on mirrors with sayings like: *I am beautiful inside and out.*
8. Affirm that your body is amazing just the way it is.
9. Walk with your head high; proud and confident in yourself as a person, not a size.
10. Don't let your size or appearance keep you from doing things you enjoy.
11. Remember that your body is not a democracy—you have the only vote.
12. Count your blessings, not your blemishes.
13. Replace the time you spend criticizing your appearance with more satisfying pursuits.
14. Every year, 98 percent of our atoms are replaced. Your body is extraordinary—respect and appreciate it!
15. Be the expert on your body. Challenge fashion magazines, cosmetic companies and weight tables.
16. Let your inner beauty and individuality shine.
17. Be your body's ally and advocate, not its enemy.
18. When you awake, thank your body for resting and rejuvenating itself so you can enjoy the day.
19. When you go to sleep, thank your body for what it helped you do throughout the day.

20. Find a method of exercise that you enjoy and do moderate amounts of it regularly. Don't do it compulsively or to lose weight—do it to feel good.
21. Think back to a time in your life when you liked and enjoyed your body. Get in touch with those memories and feelings now.
22. Look at family photos. Find the beauty, love and values in those bodies and faces. Hold them close to your heart.
23. Ask: If I had only one year to live, how important would my body image and appearance be?
24. Make a closet inventory. Do I wear clothes to hide my body or follow fashion trends in lockstep? Keep the clothes that give you feelings of pleasure, confidence and comfort.
25. Beauty is not just skin deep. It is a reflection of your whole self. Love and enjoy the person inside your skin.

A New Relationship with Our Bodies

No matter what perfectionism would have us believe or how hard we try, we cannot stop the changes that age brings to our bodies. Our lives are different from what they were two or 20 years ago, and so are our bodies. It is unhealthy to believe that we can look 25 when we're 35, 65, or 85. We need body goals and lifestyles that fit healthy reality, instead of pursuing perfection's recipe for weight loss and disaster.

I frequently encourage my patients to accept their body "as is." Recently a patient on the road to recovery added an important piece of wisdom to this phrase: "I must accept my body as is *and as it will be*." She was right—her body will continue to change, and she needs to accept that change—even if it means natural weight gain, stiffer joints, gray hair and greater wisdom.

We help ourselves accept our body "as is and as it will be" when we remember the awesome abilities of women's bodies—menstruation, ovulation, pregnancy, childbirth and lactation. The miraculous things every human body does to stay in ongoing balance and health are astounding.

- Skin replaces itself each month.
- The stomach lining re-creates itself every five days.
- Our livers reline themselves every six weeks.
- Our skeletal system replaces itself every three months.
- Within one calendar year, 98 percent of our atoms are replaced.[25]

Our "imperfect" bodies are walking, talking miracles. Be awed by their magic.

True beauty comes from the soul. To change yourself, and to conform to anyone else's standards of beauty, is to change your essence. Own who you are, and you become a truly powerful woman.[26]

Emme (Melissa Aronson)

Another simple recovery and healthy living choice is to wear clothes that fit. Tight clothes make us uncomfortable with our bodies. We have to let our clothes change as we change—an outfit that fit "perfectly" three years ago may be too small now due to the natural aging process, when middles get a bit thicker. That's a good thing, because it's a sign of how our bodies are growing to meet our changing needs!

We can even make a celebratory ritual during which a friend or kindred spirit helps us dispose of clothes that don't fit anymore. We especially need to purge our closets and psyches of those outfits we use to punish ourselves, with thoughts like "I'm a failure because I can't fit into that dress anymore." We can also take a dose of retail therapy, treating ourselves to new clothes that fit and feel great. All of it helps us enjoy our imperfect and powerful body "as is and as it will be."

Thanking our Bodies for Their Magic

Try rewarding your body for all that it does for you. Pick something from this list or come up with other ideas. Find things that feel good to your body and arrange to do them as regularly as your budget and schedule permit.

- Have a massage or some other form of therapeutic touch such as acupressure.
- Have a facial.
- Have a manicure or pedicure.
- Enjoy a sauna, steam bath, or whirlpool (if this is safe for you; your doctor can determine if these are too stressful for your heart).
- Take a class in movement, tai chi, qi gong, meditation, or mindfulness-based stress reduction.
- Practice yoga. (I recommend hatha yoga or gentle yoga; they are less stressful to the body than other kinds.)
- Experience Reiki or another form of energy medicine.

Safety in Numbers

Most people in the midst of eating or body image disorders "go it alone." Believing that we need no one or that no one else understands our problems can be seductive. It also keeps us stuck in our obsessions. Recovery and health happen when we connect with others.

We do this by joining with others, through group therapies, support groups and organizations that fight the "pursuit of perfection" and/or address other women's health issues.

Jennifer found great satisfaction and self-worth when she joined the National Eating Disorder Association. Now she volunteers in its campaigns to improve girls' and women's lives through education about body image and eating disorders. The energy, dedication and clarity of others in the organization help her to fight back against the Voice of Perfection and the impulses of her eating disorder. Many other women in recovery join these and other efforts. They find that connectedness and activism strengthen their resolve in recovery.

Avoiding Relapse

Living stressful lives in our appearance-obsessed culture presents a serious risk to women in recovery from disordered eating and body image despair. We can learn from other women's experience about how to recognize red flags that may signal a potential relapse into old, dangerous symptoms:

- more frequent obsessive thoughts about food, weight and appearance
- weighing yourself more often
- more frequent self-defeating and derogatory self-talk
- either/or, dichotomous self-perceptions (perfection/failure; thin/fat; good/bad)
- desperate need to be in control all the time
- striving for perfection and believing that the perfect weight/size/body/ grade/life will solve other problems
- feeling more competitive with peers regarding who is most attractive, thinnest, or the best dieter
- being convinced that you can restrict just for a day or purge just once without hurting yourself
- "knowing" that you are fat and unattractive even when others say you're not
- wanting to rely on no one else, proving you can handle everything on your own
- becoming more isolated and less involved with others
- choosing exercise over time with friends or other activities
- constantly checking yourself in mirrors
- being unable to look in the mirror
- making multiple clothing changes before you leave the house
- being unable to relax or to do nothing
- not sharing dark thoughts in therapy or with friends
- reverting to ritualistic eating habits

- drinking large quantities of water, alcohol, coffee, diet soda, or tea to fill you up and cope with hunger
- feeling more hopeless and depressed, but not telling anyone
- avoiding therapy or other relationships that help to keep you honest.

If you recognize these warning signs in your life, you are on the road to relapse and you need to take a detour. Even a few red flags show your vulnerability and the importance of addressing the shape of your inner life so that you do not succumb to the dangerous cycle of basing your worth on the shape of your external body.

> As long as our orientation is toward perfection or success, we will never learn about unconditional friendship with ourselves, nor will we find compassion.[27]
>
> Pema Chödrön

Getting well is only the first step in recovery. Staying well and embracing life make up all the other steps. Those steps include incorporating positive attitudes and activities into everyday life.

Fortunately, women's experience reveals simple, healthy strategies that work if taken seriously and practiced daily.

- Do something that you love for at least 10 minutes.
- Eat foods that you enjoy.
- Wear clothes that fit and feel good.
- Loosen up when feeling rigid or perfectionistic.
- Give yourself some compliments.
- Say yes and say no; don't just let life happen to you.
- Be mindful and take time to reflect.
- Do nice things for your body.
- Count your blessings.
- Make a daily gratitude list at least five items long.
- Stay connected with positive people in your life.
- Declare: "My body is not a democracy—I'm the only one who gets a vote." Believe this with all your heart, and then act on it daily.

Most of all, we need to find hope in our search for recovery. A woman with an eating or body image disorder needs to believe that she can in fact recover (because that's true). She also needs to call on resources and people to keep going and growing. The words of this Tibetan Prayer capture what we need to move forward and stay well:

> May I be at peace.
> My heart remain open.
> May I know the beauty of my own true nature.
> May I be healed.[28]

Embracing Ourselves

Writing about her recovery from bulimia and body image obsessions, actress Yeardly Smith (the voice of Lisa on *The Simpsons*) says she used to see her body as her enemy:

> I have things more in perspective now. [For example,] I don't regret my plastic surgery, but I do regret feeling at the time that I couldn't live without having it. I've learned to accept who I am, thank God, because there is so much energy that goes into that self-loathing of "how come my hips aren't a size 36" or whatever. All of those feelings of failure are completely in my own head. I finally get it.[29]

No matter where you were when you started this book, you now know that the desire for perfection or a perfect body is not an immutable force of nature. In fact, it is not natural. It is not even a true desire.

I hope that you are now more convinced of the need for every one of us to embrace ourselves fully. Even if you're that rare woman who never in her life had a bad body-image day, your role is just as important as anyone else's.

Whether or not we have an eating disorder or body image problem, we can help one another by challenging the pursuit of perfection, refusing to speak the language of fat, and showing one another that the shape we are in is not determined by the shape of our bodies.

> To believe that you must hide all the parts of you that are broken, out of fear that someone else is incapable of loving what is less than perfect, is to believe that sunlight is incapable of entering a broken window and illuminating a dark room.[30]
>
> Marc Chernoff

Let the light in. I am not my body. You are not your body. Each of our bodies is an important, lovable vehicle, but it is not the journey or the destination. Nor is it our enemy.

Your imperfect body is worth respecting and appreciating, no matter how it is shaped or how you think it looks. Even more important, your imperfect life is worth respecting and appreciating. So let's agree to embrace our bodies and our lives—along with the bodies and lives of every other woman.

Notes

1   *What If God Were One of Us? A Cry to Awaken, New Revelations* (Bloomington, IN: iUniverse, 2011) p. 192.

2   Margery Williams, *The Velveteen Rabbit* (New York: Avon, 1975) pp. 16–17.

3 "Listening to Shame." *TED Talks* presentation, published March 16, 2012. See www.youtube.com/watch?v=psN1DORYYV0&feature=youtu.be (retrieved August 26, 2015).

4 "Diary." *London Review of Books*, 35 (3) pp. 34–35. See www.lrb.co.uk/v35/n03/rebecca-solnit/diary (retrieved August 26, 2015).

5 Thich Nhat Hanh, *Peace Is Every Step* (New York: Bantam, 1991).

6 *A Woman of Her Tribe* (New York: Atheneum, 1990) p. 51.

7 Ibid.

8 *Arriving at Your Own Door: 108 Lessons in Mindfulness* (New York: Hyperion, 2007) p. 7.

9 "Stop 'Shoulding' Yourself to Death!" *Psychology Today*, posted April 3, 2013. See www.psychologytoday.com/blog/inviting-monkey-tea/201304/stop-shoulding-yourself-death-0 (retrieved August 26, 2015).

10 Demosthenes B. Panagiotakos, Christina Chrysohoou, Gerasimos Siasos, Konstantinos Zisimos, John Skoumas, Christos Pitsavos and Christodoulos Stefanadis (2011) "Sociodemographic and lifestyle statistics of oldest old people (>80 years) living in Ikaria island: The Ikaria study." *Cardiology Research and Practice* Volume 2011, Article ID 679187, 7 pages.

11 *Wildfire: Igniting the She/Volution* (Wildfire Books, 1990) p. 219.

12 University of Michigan Panel Study on Income Dynamics (2008) "Chore Wars: Men, Women and Housework." National Science Foundation, posted April 28, 2008. See www.nsf.gov/discoveries/disc_images.jsp?cntn_id=111458 (retrieved August 26, 2015).

13 Adapted from Stacie Stukin (2003) "The Anti-Drug for Anxiety." *Yoga Journal*, March–April, 2003, 108–113.

14 See Thomas F. Schwartz (2003) "'You Can Fool All of the People' Lincoln Never Said That." *For the People: A Newsletter of the Abraham Lincoln Association*, 5 (4), 1. See www.abrahamlincolnassociation.org/Newsletters/5-4.pdf (retrieved August 26, 2015).

15 Linda Bacon and Lucy Aphramor, *Body Respect: What Conventional Health Books Get Wrong, Leave Out, and Just Plain Fail to Understand about Weight* (Dallas, TX: BenBella Books, 2014).

16 Glenn A. Gaesser, *Big Fat Lies* (Carlsbad, CA: Gürze Books, 2002).

17 Linda Bacon and Lucy Aphramor (2011) "Weight science: Evaluating the evidence for a paradigm shift." *Nutrition Journal*, 10 (9); doi:10.1186/1475-2891-10-9. See www.nutritionj.com/content/10/1/9 (retrieved January 13, 2016).

18 *Life, the Truth, and Being Free* (Port Washington, NY: A Better Today Publishing, 2009) p. 147.

19 Bacon and Aphramor, 2014.

20 E.g., Mark V. Roehling, Patricia V. Roehling and Shaun Pichler (2007) "The relationships between body weight and perceived weight-related employment discrimination: The role of sex and race." *Journal of Vocational Behavior*, 71 (2), 300–318. See www.researchgate.net/profile/Patricia_Roehling/publication/222821227 (retrieved January 13, 2016).

21 Roberta R. Friedman and Rebecca M. Puhl, *Weight Bias: A Social Justice Issue: A Policy Brief* (New Haven, CT: Yale Rudd Center for Food Policy and Obesity, 2012). See www.uconnruddcenter.org/resources/upload/docs/what/reports/Rudd_Policy_Brief_Weight_Bias.pdf (retrieved August 26, 2015).

22 See www.marketresearch.com/Marketdata-Enterprises-Inc-v416/Weight-Loss-Status-Forecast-8016030/ (retrieved August 26, 2015).

23 See www.marketsandmarkets.com/PressReleases/global-market-for-weight-loss-worth-$726-billion-by-2014.asp (retrieved August 26, 2015).

24 Adapted from Maine, *Body Wars: Making Peace with Women's Bodies* (Carlsbad, CA: Gürze Books, 2000).
25 See Deepak Chopra, *Ageless Body, Timeless Mind* (New York: Harmony, 1993).
26 Personal communication with Margo Maine, September, 2015. The most prominent plus-size model for decades, Emme advocates for positive body image and appreciation of women's true beauty and value. She has been named one of *People* magazine's "50 Most Beautiful People" (1994 and 1999), *Glamour* magazine's "Woman of the Year" (1997) and a "Most Important Women in America" (1999) and a "Most Fascinating Women of the Year" (1997) by *Ladies' Home Journal*.
27 "Signs of Spiritual Progress" on Lion's Roar: Buddhist Wisdom for Our Time, posted July 18, 2014. See www.lionsroar.com/how-to-meditate-pema-chodron-on-signs-of-spiritual-progress/ (retrieved September 16, 2015).
28 Source unknown, shared by Carolyn Costin.
29 "After 25 Years, Yeardley Smith—the Voice of TV's Sax-Playing Sage, Lisa Simpson—Scores a Victory Over Bulimia and Self-Doubt." *People*, 61 (16) April 26, 2004, p. 100.
30 "12 Things You Should Know for Sure." Posted October 26, 2012. See www.marcandangel.com/2012/10/26/12-things-you-should-know-for-sure/ (retrieved November 12, 2015).

Appendix

Resources for Eating Disorders and Body Image Despair

Our website www.womenpersuingperfection.com has easy links to all of these websites and books, as well as other information and resources.

Websites

www.about-face-org About-Face promotes positive self-esteem in women of all ages through media education, outreach and activism.

www.aedweb.org The Academy for Eating Disorders is a professional organization that provides training and education to clinicians and dedicates itself to improving the research, treatment and prevention of eating disorders.

www.anad.org The National Association of Anorexia Nervosa and Related Disorders provides eating disorders information, referrals, education and support groups.

www.andreasvoice.org Critical and helpful information for sufferers and their families from a moving website dedicated to a young woman who died from bulimia.

www.bedaonline.com Home of the Binge Eating Disorder Association, a national organization focused on recognition, prevention and treatment of BED and associated weight stigma.

www.thebodypositive.org The Body Positive teaches people of all ages how to overcome conflicts with their bodies so they can lead happier, more productive lives.

www.cswd.org The Council on Size and Weight Discrimination advocates for people of all sizes and provides education and information on fairness, weight bias and media images.

www.eatingdisorderscoalition.org The Eating Disorders Coalition for Research, Policy, and Action advocates with US federal policymakers and legislators for the recognition of eating disorders as a major public health problem.

www.edcatalogue.com The respected Gürze-Slucore organization's website is both a bookstore and a resource for information about eating disorders.

www.edreferral.com The Eating Disorder Referral and Information Center has free information and referral lists for treatment of eating disorders.

www.healthyweight.net The Healthy Weight Network provides up-to-date information on eating and weight research and diet quackery, and promotes the Health At Every Size (HAES) movement.

www.iaedp.com The International Association of Eating Disorders Professionals provides education and training to professionals.

www.joekelly.org My co-author's site provides excellent resources for fathers, stepfathers and other men in families, coaching for family members of someone suffering from eating disorders and on his consulting for health professionals.

www.mentalhealthscreening.org This organization sponsors screening, education and outreach programs for eating disorders through the National Eating Disorder Screening Project.

www.mwsg.org The website for my professional practice, Maine & Weinstein Specialty Group, provides helpful information and links to other sites.

www.nationaleatingdisorders.org The National Eating Disorders Association is the largest US organization providing educational materials, programs and referral information. NEDA also sponsors the annual Eating Disorders Awareness Week each February. A great resource for the public and professionals.

www.theselflovediet.org Includes an online course to lead you towards self-acceptance, body acceptance, healing and self-love.

www.theelisaproject.com The Elisa Project sponsors education and outreach programs in the Dallas Metroplex.

Books

Berg, Francie, *Women Afraid To Eat: Breaking Free in Today's Weight-Obsessed World*. Hettinger, ND: Healthy Weight Network, 2001.

Borysenko, Joan, *A Woman's Book of Life: The Biology, Psychology, and Spirituality of the Feminine Life Cycle*. New York: Riverhead Books, 1996.

Brumberg, Joan Jacobs, *The Body Project: An Intimate History of American Girls*. New York: Random House, 1997.

Chernin, Kim, *The Hungry Self: Women, Eating and Identity*. New York: First Harper Perennial, 1994.

Costin, Carolyn, *100 Questions and Answers About Eating Disorders*. Boston: Jones & Bartlett, 2007.

Costin, Carolyn, *The Eating Disorder Sourcebook: A Comprehensive Guide to the Causes, Treatment, and Prevention of Eating Disorders (3rd Edition)*. New York: McGraw-Hill, 2006.

Costin, Carolyn and Grabb, Gwen Schubert, *8 Keys to Recovery from an Eating Disorder: Effective Strategies from Therapeutic Practice and Personal Experience*. New York: W. W. Norton, 2011.

Costin, Carolyn and Kelly, Joe (Eds.), *Yoga and Eating Disorders: Ancient Healing for a Modern Illness*. New York: Routledge, 2016.

Domar, Alice D. and Dreher, Henry, *Self-Nurture: Learning to Care for Yourself As Effectively As You Care for Everyone Else*. New York: Viking, 2000.

Durek, Judith, *Circle of Stones: Woman's Journey to Herself*. San Diego, CA: LuraMedia, 1999.

Durek, Judith, *I Sit Listening to the Wind: Woman's Encounter within Herself*. San Diego, CA: LuraMedia, 1993.

Fallon, Patricia, Katzman, Melanie A. and Wooley, Susan C., *Feminist Perspectives on Eating Disorders*. New York: Guilford, 1993.

Fodor, Viola, *Desperately Seeking Self: An Inner Guidebook for People with Eating Problems*. Carlsbad, CA: Gürze Books, 1997.

Freedman, Rita, *Bodylove: Learning to Like Our Looks and Ourselves.* Carlsbad, CA: Gürze Books, 2002.

Friedman, Sandra, *Body Thieves.* Vancouver, BC: Salal Books, 2002.

Friedman, Sandra, *When Girls Feel Fat.* Buffalo, NY: Firefly Books, 2000.

Gaesser, Glenn A. *Big Fat Lies: The Truth About Your Weight and Your Health.* Carlsbad, CA: Gürze Books, 2002.

Hall, Lindsey, *The Ritteroo Journal for Eating Disorders Recovery.* Carlsbad, CA: Gürze Books, 2013.

Hall, Lindsey (Ed.), *Full Lives: Women Who Have Freed Themselves from Food and Weight Obsession.* Carlsbad, CA: Gürze Books, 1993.

Hall, Lindsey and Cohn, Leigh, *Bulimia: A Guide to Recovery.* Carlsbad, CA: Gürze Books, 1999.

Hall, Lindsey and Ostroff, Monika, *Anorexia Nervosa: A Guide to Recovery.* Carlsbad, CA: Gürze Books, 1999.

Hutchinson, Marcia Germaine, *Transforming Body Image.* Freedom, CA: The Crossing Press, 1985.

Johnston, Anita, *Eating In the Light of the Moon.* Carlsbad, CA: Gürze Books, 2000.

Kabat-Zinn, Jon, *Coming to Our Senses: Healing Ourselves and the World Through Mindfulness.* New York: Hyperion, 2005.

Kabat-Zinn, Jon, *Full Catastrophe Living: Using the Wisdom of Your Body and Mind to Face Stress, Pain, and Illness.* New York: Delacorte, 1990.

Kabat-Zinn, Jon, *Wherever You Go, There You Are.* New York: Hyperion, 1994.

Kearney-Cooke, Ann and Issacs, Florence, *Change Your Mind, Change Your Body: Feeling Good About Your Body and Your Self After 40.* New York: Atria Books, 2004.

Kelly, Joe, *Dads & Daughters®: How to Inspire, Support and Understand Your Daughter.* New York: Broadway, 2003.

Kilbourne, Jean, *Can't Buy My Love: How Advertising Changes the Way We Think and Feel.* New York: Simon and Schuster, 2000.

Kingsbury, Kathleen Burns and Williams, Mary Ellen, *Weight Wisdom: Affirmations to Free You from Food and Body Concerns.* New York: Brunner/Routledge, 2003.

Knapp, Caroline. *Appetites: Why Women Want.* New York: Counterpoint, 2002.

Koenig, Karen R., *The Rules of "Normal" Eating: A Commonsense Approach for Dieters, Overeaters, Undereaters, Emotional Eaters, and Everyone in Between.* Carlsbad, CA: Gürze Books. 2005.

Lerner, Harriet, *The Dance of Anger: A Woman's Guide to Changing Patterns of Intimate Relationships.* New York: Harper Collins, 1985.

Maine, Margo, *Father Hunger: Fathers, Daughters and the Pursuit of Thinness.* Carlsbad, CA: Gürze Books, 2004.

Maine, Margo, *Body Wars: Making Peace with Women's Bodies.* Carlsbad, CA: Gürze Books, 2000.

Maine, Margo, Davis, William and Shure, Jane (Eds.), *Effective Clinical Practice in the Treatment of Eating Disorders: The Heart of the Matter.* New York: Routledge, 2009.

Maine, Margo, McGilley, Beth Hartman and Bunnell, Douglas (Eds.), *Treatment of Eating Disorders: Bridging the Research-Practice Gap.* London, UK: Elsevier, 2010.

Manheim, Camryn, *Wake Up, I'm Fat!* New York: Broadway Books, 1999.

Minero, Michelle, *The Self-Love Diet: The Only Diet that Works.* Sausalito, CA: Phoenix Century Press, 2013.

Nasser, Mervat, Katzman, Melanie A. and Gordon, Richard A. (Eds.), *Eating Disorders and Cultures in Transition.* New York: Brunner-Routledge, 2001.

Northrup, Christiane, *Women's Bodies, Women's Wisdom: Creating Physical and Emotional Health and Healing.* New York: Bantam Books, 2010.

Northrup, Christiane, *The Wisdom of Menopause: Creating Physical and Emotional Health During the Change.* New York: Bantam, 2012.

Northrup, Christiane, *Goddesses Never Age: The Secret Prescription for Radiance, Vitality, and Well-Being.* Carlsbad, CA: Hay House, 2015.

Piran, Niva, Levine, Michael P. and Steiner-Adair, Catherine (Eds.), *Preventing Eating Disorders: A Handbook of Interventions and Special Challenges.* Philadelphia, PA: Taylor & Francis, Inc., 1999.

Rabinor, Judith Ruskay, *A Starving Madness: Tales of Hunger, Hope, and Healing in Psychotherapy.* Carlsbad, CA: Gürze Books, 2002.

Radcliffe, Rebecca, *Dance Naked In Your Living Room: Handling Stress and Finding Joy.* Minneapolis, MN: Ease Publications, 1997.

Radcliffe, Rebecca, *Body Prayers: Finding Body Peace.* Minneapolis, MN: Ease Publications, 1999.

Radcliffe, Rebecca, *Hot Flashes, Chocolate Sauce, & Rippled Thighs: Women's Wisdom, Wellness, and Body Gratitude.* Minneapolis, MN: Ease Publications, 2004.

Roth, Geneen, *When Food Is Love: Exploring the Relationship between Eating and Intimacy.* New York: Plume Books, 1991.

Sarasohn, Lisa, *The Woman's Belly Book: Finding Your Treasure Within.* Asheville, NC: Self Health Education, 2003.

Steinem, Gloria, *Revolution from Within: A Book of Self-Esteem.* Boston: Little Brown, 1992.

Waterhouse, Debra, *Like Mother, Like Daughter: How Women Are Influenced by Their Mother's Relationship with Food and How to Break the Pattern.* New York: Hyperion, 1997.

Thomas, Jennifer J. and Schaefer, Jenni, *Almost Anorexic: Is My (or My Loved One's) Relationship with Food a Problem?* Center City, MN: Hazelden, 2013.

Wolf, Naomi, *The Beauty Myth: How Images of Beauty are Used Against Women.* New York: Perennial, 2002.

Zerbe, Kathryn J., *Integrated Treatment of Eating Disorders: Beyond the Body Betrayed.* New York: Norton, 2008.

Index